Praise for *Hope*

"Completing the inspiring story that her father began, Jamie weaves a narrative of faith and possibility in the shadow of a dire prognosis. A valuable and well-told account of a family's courageous journey."

—Kevin Patrick Allen
Documentary Filmmaker

"Jamie has an indomitable spirit, which she obviously gets from her father! This book is an inspiring labor of love and source of hope for cancer patients and their families."

—Michael Veltri
Leadership Expert, Best-Selling Author,
Marine Veteran, Cancer Survivor, and Keynote Speaker

"A powerful and heartwarming read offering hope and inspiration to all."

—Chuck Carroll
Weight Loss Champion and *The Exam Room* Podcast Host

"A powerful and inspiring journey of faith, love, and family intimately woven with joy, grief, strength, and loss; a sharing that will connect with each reader's heart and soul. Through Jimmy and Jamie Blanco, I have learned resilience and I have been given a gift. This book is a must read!"

—Roselle P. O'Brien
MA, MFA, LMHC, LCMHC, REAT, REACE

Hope for the Hopeless

Hope for the Hopeless

How One Man Fought the World's Deadliest Brain Tumor on His Terms and Won

Jimmy Blanco & Jamie Blanco

BOOKLOGIX®
Alpharetta, GA

ISBN: 978-1-6653-0371-2 - Paperback
eISBN: 978-1-6653-0372-9 - ebook

Library of Congress Control Number: 2022907580

∞This paper meets the requirements of ANSI/NISO Z39.48-1992 (Permanence of Paper)

Cover art: rebecacovers
Cover photo: Medical x-ray of the human brain by merrydolla
Photos of Jimmy Blanco provided by Elizabeth Blanco

Scripture quotations marked "NKJV" are taken from the New King James Version®. Copyright © 1982 by Thomas Nelson. Used by permission. All rights reserved.

060122

This book is dedicated to Jesus Christ, who found it in His heart to guide me and heal me of my "incurable" cancer for many years. I thank the Lord for allowing me the honor of being an instrument of His healing. Thank you for healing me and for giving me the strength and the faith I needed to fight my cancer effectively. Thank you for giving me the inspiration to write this book and pass on to others the secrets of nature.

To my family, who stood behind me.
To my father and mother, whom I love dearly.
To my lovely wife, Elizabeth, who cared for me.
To my beautiful children, Jamie, Jimmy Jr., and Jason.
To all the wonderful people who prayed for my recovery.
—Jimmy Blanco

Contents

Preface

This is the true story of my fight with one of the world's deadliest cancers. It's a story filled with miracles. I was given three months to live if I did not take radiation and chemotherapy treatments for my "incurable" brain cancer. I ventured out alone with no help, but with God's guidance, I was led in the right direction and found what appears to be an effective natural treatment for my so-called incurable disease.

I refused to die just because the doctors said I was supposed to. I didn't have time to die; instead, I would be very busy trying to prove them wrong. I do not take no for an answer. I believe it was because of my character that God chose me for this mission. The doctors, with all their PhDs and degrees, threw their hands up, first in surrender and then in disbelief. Their explanation: it must be a misdiagnosis. Unfortunately for that theory, I had my brain tissue matched with a cheek sample for DNA analysis. The odds were one in fifty-two million that it was not mine.

They warned me and pressured me, "You'll be dead in three months." I was so confident that God would guide me in the right direction that I documented everything I did from day one. Seventeen months later I was not only alive but my deadly brain tumor, a glioblastoma multiforme grade IV, could not be found on an MRI.

That's when I decided to begin writing this book.

I have experienced many miracles in this time, from surviving a grand mal seizure behind the wheel of my van to being brought back from the brink by my Lord in an emergency room. My inspiration for writing this book is to be able to help the people whom the doctors cannot. I want to help the hopeless cases out there like me. My mission in life was just beginning while the doctors were thinking that it was over. My mission was to stay alive to write this book and get the word out.

The word is this: there is "Hope for the Hopeless," and a cure for the incurable. I was also told that I would be the first person with my diagnosis to survive long enough to write a book. I feel I owe it to the ones who come after me.

The healthcare system and the medical establishment are going to have to change in the very near future.

After contacting and talking to many doctors to find answers, I now understand why there have not been any major break-throughs in the fight against cancer. No one in the medical field has been the least bit interested in finding out why I have done so well without radiation or chemotherapy.

They haven't asked themselves, "Could there be a scientific reason why I have not had a recurrent tumor?" No, they just shrug it off as a fluke, and they all have given me a story of the one person who also beat the odds.

Why should they only have one story?

Why can't they have a million stories to tell?

Why should I be the exception instead of the rule?

If they were interested in finding advances in the possible cure and/or management of glioblastoma multiforme, they would be beating my doors down and my phone would be ringing off the hook. They would be trying to find out what I have done differently than everyone else. Why am I alive with no tumor growth while others are dying?

They will not believe that the cure could possibly be as simple as taking supplements, changing one's lifestyle and eating habits, and harnessing the power of your God-given mind.

The truth will emerge and people will begin to demand more answers. The doctors were playing God, but I turned to the real God and asked Him to guide me to the truth and a treatment. He did, and this is my story.

Jimmy Blanco

Introduction

A t the time of his death in 2003, my father, Jimmy Blanco, was one of the longest-living survivors of a glioblastoma multiforme (GBM) grade IV brain tumor. And he did it without traditional medicine.

GBMs famously claimed the lives of John McCain, Ted Kennedy, and Joe Biden's son Beau, all of whom had access to the best that medical science currently has to offer. And this terrible disease continues to ravage those who fall victim to it, with instances continuing to grow globally.

The GBM is the most devastating and deadly brain tumor in the world and typically kills within several months without treatment. The National Foundation for Cancer Research reports GBMs account for 45 percent of all malignant brain tumors, and it remains unclear what causes these cancerous tumors and whether genetics or environmental factors play a role.[1]

They are notoriously treacherous to treat because their tendrils invade tissue rapidly, mutating and spreading with gut-wrenching speed. Even with surgery, these tumors recur aggressively and quickly. GBMs do not quit. But there has been progress since the time of my father's illness in the '90s and early 2000s.

Life expectancies have now been extended to an average of about fifteen months in the United States with newer traditional

---

[1] "Cancer Facts & Figures 2021," American Cancer Society, 2021. https://www.cancer.org/research/cancer-facts-statistics/all-cancer-facts-figures/cancer-facts-figures-2021.html.

therapies.[2] According to the Central Brain Tumor Registry, only 7 percent of patients survive five years after diagnosis, up from 4 percent.[3] Even so, there have been several glioblastoma super-survivors associated with the newest clinical trials. I will detail those exciting developments a little later on.

But at the time of my father's original diagnosis in October of 1995, there was little hope he would live longer than three months, maybe a few weeks more with traditional interventions.

My father lived *eight years*. He never did chemotherapy, radiation, clinical trials, or other mainstream treatments other than surgery. Instead, he relied on natural medicine, nutrition, mental focus techniques like visualization, and his unshakable faith.

He was a miracle, and so are you.

Life was breathed into your cells. You think and love and live in an infinite universe of seeming nothingness, and yet here you are.

When you learn biology, you quickly discover that the fact that anyone is alive at all is a monumental achievement. The processes in your body must be in such precise harmony to function that it is staggering to imagine. The tiniest imbalances mean certain death, and yet it all operates without a single thought from you.

Nature, when left to its own devices, balances itself. Ecosystems flourish in harmony and this world goes on, miracle upon the miracle of life. That leads me to my second favorite passage of the Bible.

In Matthew, Jesus says, "Look at the birds of the air, for they neither sow nor reap nor gather into barns; yet your heavenly

---

[2] Derek R. Johnson, Heather E. Leeper, and Joon H. Uhm, "Glioblastoma survival in the United States improved after Food and Drug Administration approval of bevacizumab: A population-based analysis," Cancer 119, no. 19 (2013): 3489–3495. https://acsjournals.onlinelibrary.wiley.com/doi/full/10.1002/cncr.28259.

[3] Kimberly D. Miller et al., "Brain and Other Central Nervous System Tumor Statistics, 2021," American Cancer Society Journals, American Cancer Society, August 24, 2021. https://acsjournals.onlinelibrary.wiley.com/doi/10.3322/caac.21693.

Father feeds them. Are you not of more value than they? . . . So why do you worry about clothing? Consider the lilies of the field, how they grow: they neither toil nor spin; and yet I say to you that even Solomon in all his glory was not arrayed like one of these.

"Now if God so clothes the grass of the field, which today is, and tomorrow is thrown into the oven, will He not much more clothe you, O you of little faith?" (Matthew 6:26–34 (NKJV)).

If this is my second favorite, what is my first favorite passage of the Bible, you might ask?

That would be how Jesus's first miracle came about because he was at a wedding that ran out of wine. His mother, Mary, says, in essence, "Jesus, come over here and make with the God powers," and Jesus answers in what I imagine to be an exasperated voice, "Woman, my time has not yet come." Mary, who was not having any of it, replied to the effect of, "Don't 'woman' me, I am your mother and your mother is telling you to make with the water-to-wine trick because we have a party to save." Jesus looks up to heaven, where God shrugs his shoulders and says, "Listen to your mother." First, save the party, then mankind's souls. The relatability of the story makes me grin uncontrollably every time.

My father's story is a bit different.

This is the story of my father's miracle and how in his unerring faith he was provided for. This is our family's testimonial written over the course of more than twenty years.

I'll start where it began for me.

I was nine years old when my father got sick.

We lived in a small, two-story townhouse in Miami, Florida, with a long backyard that backed up to a tollbooth behind the Florida Turnpike. We could see Florida International University and the National Hurricane Center across the highway from our covered terrace. The tollbooth bell sounded all day long from people blowing through it without paying, and the sound of ambulances whipping up and down the highway to the nearby hospital was constant. But it was always lush and green and warm outside.

My father built us a swing set, and at the very end of the yard, we grew bananas and mangos, though it seemed like hurricanes always blew the banana trees down every time they would finally give fruit. He tried to give us everything he never had growing up in the '60s and '70s on the streets of Bayonne, New Jersey, to poor immigrant parents.

My paternal grandparents came to this country from Cuba in the mid-1950s because of the economic oppression of the Batista regime. They came in pursuit of the American Dream and a better life for their children. As a baby, my father lived in a tiny, rundown apartment in New Jersey. He had no crib, so instead, they put him in a dresser drawer to sleep. There, he survived being nearly eaten by rats in the middle of the night. Horrified for his baby and unable to provide for his young family, my grandfather sent my grandmother, my father, and his two older siblings back to Cuba for several years while he stayed in the US and sent money back home. When Castro rose to power, they escaped again.

My father's early life was seemingly all struggles. As a kid, he survived a brick to the head from a neighborhood bully. As a teen and young adult, he lived through race riots, neighborhood gangs, and other challenges I can't even imagine. He spent time in the army and navy before moving to Miami. Now, as a parent, his own kids would want for nothing.

I lived with my parents, my two younger brothers, my paternal grandparents, and my teenage uncle Lazaro. It was a messy, chaotic house full of love.

It was the day before my mother's birthday, October 26, 1995, and my father was going in for another long shift at Miami Children's Hospital, where he worked as a respiratory therapist. I sometimes wonder how many lives he would be saving today during the coronavirus pandemic had he lived this long. My father took as many double shifts as he could so that all three of his children could attend a safe private school. I remember being sad that I didn't see him as much around that time because he was always at work.

It was not because I missed him that nine-year-old me begged him to stay that night. I *knew* something terrible was going to happen. The feeling overwhelmed me. I cried for him not to go, to stay home and rest. I told him I had a bad feeling and that he shouldn't leave. I pushed hard, but he said he had to go. He walked out the door in his blue scrubs, kissing me under his thick manicured mustache and huge, square '90s glasses, shaking his thick, black, curly hair with an expression that said, *Don't worry about me, kid.*

We woke up to the news that Daddin (our name for him) had been in a car accident and had to have surgery. Somehow, that didn't scare me. I thought that since he made it to the hospital and the doctors were taking care of him, everything was going to be okay. What I didn't know was that he had suffered a massive grand mal seizure behind the wheel and he was undergoing life-saving surgery to remove a golf ball-sized tumor from his brain.

"I told you I had a bad feeling," I told my mother. She and my grandmother whispered about it in Spanish.

At the time, my brothers and I went to a private Christian school called Tropical Christian School in the heart of horse country. It was one of the reasons my father worked so hard, so he could give his three kids, whom he loved more fiercely than life itself, a good education in a safe environment. Where we lived, in Southwest Miami-Dade near Eighth Street, was not exactly the best area for schools.

I remember my mother taking me to TCS and making me wait outside the office while she talked to the principal. I remember just being happy to get out of school for a few days, perfectly oblivious to the seismic tragedy beginning to unfold for my family.

There was a day I remember distinctly: The Friday after returning to class, we had a schoolwide church service, and the principal asked everyone to pray for my father who was in a car accident. My friends turned to me with looks of concern and confusion and asked, "Your father was in an accident?" And I just smiled and said, "Yup!" I wasn't worried. I had no idea.

When we went to see him in the hospital, they had shaved his head and he had a huge half-moon scar on his head. He couldn't walk, but he still joked with us and made us laugh, and we took silly pictures in the hospital room. I wasn't worried. I had no idea.

A few weeks later, my father was home alone with us while my mother was at work. She was a medical transcriptionist at a nearby hospital. Daddin was still recovering and trying to sleep. My brothers and I were screaming and fighting when he got frustrated. He pulled us together and told us that he needed us to be quiet because Daddin was very sick.

And then he screamed at us (or it felt like screaming because he was crying and I'd never heard a more frightening sound in my life), "I have cancer!"

I don't know what my brothers did; I vaguely remember them crying. J. J. was eight and Jason was six, so I don't even know if they understood what it meant. But I did. I remember calling my mother, who was at work, and screaming at her, demanding to know why she didn't tell me.

Then I locked myself in my room.

I cried and prayed harder than I have in my entire life. I was in this state for at least an hour. I called up to God in my little voice and I begged Him not to take Daddin away from us. I begged Him to make me sick instead, to let us keep our Daddin. I had an almost out-of-body experience looking down on myself from the ceiling as I cried between my bed and the sliding glass window.

I believe there was no small power in that prayer, and in all the other prayers from family, friends, and our school community.

Daddin was thirty-six years old, married with three young kids, and the doctors had just given him three months to live.

But from day one he rejected the doctors' death sentence for him.

He was walking with my mother in the mall trying to figure out what they were going to do when he stumbled upon a book called *Sharks Don't Get Cancer* by Dr. William Lane. The book claimed that shark cartilage could slow or halt the growth of blood vessels that feed tumors.

He began taking BeneFin shark cartilage and other natural supplements, rejecting all traditional treatments at the time because they did not offer him hope for survival or quality of life.

Because of his decision, doctors and surgeons refused to treat him. They told him not to talk to other cancer patients. He was turned down from several clinical trials because my father refused to stop taking his supplements. Nearly a year later, doctors wrote him off as having been misdiagnosed, so my father had his samples retested multiple times. They always came back the same: glioblastoma multiforme grade IV.

During this time, the FDA was trying to shut down the production of the product he believed was keeping him alive. I remember his anxiety of not knowing if he'd be able to put in his next order for shark cartilage.

Clinical trials about the effectiveness of shark cartilage were, and still are, woefully incomplete.

The Research

It has since been established that, yes, sharks do in fact get cancer, but despite the issue with the title, the benefits of shark cartilage cannot be completely dismissed.

Shark cartilage became a sensation back in 1993, making a splash on an international scale when Dr. William Lane published the results of a study conducted in Cuba on twenty-nine patients with advanced terminal cancers. In an interview in Shark Cartilage Exchange, Dr. Lane said, after nearly three years of treatment with pure shark cartilage, "[Fourteen] out of 29 terminal cancer patients were completely well and cancer-free."[4] Nine of the patients died of cancer and six others died of other causes. He was featured twice on *60*

---

[4] I. William Lane, PhD, Shark cartilage therapy: A Personal History of Its Development, p.2–7.

Minutes, leading to a huge burst of interest in this seeming miracle treatment.

Lane's studies, however, were not controlled studies; his results were never published in peer-reviewed journals and he was criticized for his methodology. The National Cancer Institute's Division of Cancer Treatment called the data "incomplete and unimpressive."[5]

Even so, millions of people began taking the supplements, spurring researchers to begin trials of their own.

The way shark cartilage purports to work is by limiting the growth of new blood vessels that feed the tumors—in other words, the inhibition of angiogenesis. Some studies have observed anti-angiogenesis properties in shark cartilage. In an article published in the journal *Science* in 1983 researchers found, "Shark cartilage contains a substance that strongly inhibits the growth of new blood vessels toward solid tumors, thereby restricting tumor growth." It goes on to conclude, "The abundance of this factor in shark cartilage, in contrast to cartilage from mammalian sources, may make sharks an ideal source of the inhibitor and may help to explain the rarity of neoplasms in these animals."[6]

Several animal studies used rabbits that had pellets containing basic fibroblast growth factor (bFGF) surgically implanted into their corneas to induce angiogenesis. They demonstrated that, "in the rabbit, oral shark cartilage appears to produce systemic levels of angiogenesis inhibitors that can exert their effect at the cornea."[7]

―――――――――――――

[5] J. Matthews, "Media Feeds Frenzy over Shark Cartilage as Cancer Treatment." Journal of the National Cancer Institute 85, no. 15 (1993): 1190–91. https://doi.org/10.1093/jnci/85.15.1190.

[6] A. Lee and R. Langer, "Shark Cartilage Contains Inhibitors of Tumor Angiogenesis," Science 221 (1983): 1185–87. https://doi.org/10.1126/science.6193581.

[7] R. P. González et al., "Demonstration of Inhibitory Effect of Oral Shark Cartilage on Basic Fibroblast Growth Factor-Induced Angiogenesis in the Rabbit Cornea," Biological & Pharmaceutical Bulletin 24, no. 2 (2001): 151–54. https://doi.org/10.1248/bpb.24.151.

However, it has been far more difficult to observe anti-angiogenesis in action in human patients.

Of the numerous clinical trials investigating the effectiveness of shark cartilage on cancer over the years, none have been conclusive.

The National Center for Biotechnological Information of the National Institutes of Health and ClinicalTrials.gov are great resources for seeing current and previous trials that have been conducted and their outcomes.

Most if not all of the shark cartilage trials, regardless of the type of cancer, were conducted on pretreated patients with advanced disease in combination with traditional therapies like chemo and radiation.

Proponents of shark cartilage strongly believe that the toxicity of treatments like chemo and radiation destroys the efficacy of shark cartilage.

The US National Cancer Institute conducted a large, two-year, randomized, double-blind study of the powdered BeneFin shark cartilage as a complementary treatment, again, alongside chemo and radiation, to see if it improved outcomes and well-being in breast and colorectal cancer patients. The study was shut down after two years when it became clear that the shark cartilage was not benefiting patients, but causing gastrointestinal issues in a number of the study participants.[8]

There has been some question as to whether the material of the powdered shark cartilage is able to be broken down and absorbed properly by the body, but there has been some promising anti-cancer activity observed in level III clinical trials of the liquid form of shark cartilage.

The liquid shark cartilage extract, called AE-941, has been shown to stop the growth of certain cancer cells in lab tests, as well as block the formation of new blood vessels. But AE-941 has not

---

[8] D. R. Miller, G. T. Anderson, J. J. Stark, J. L. Granick, and D. Richardson, "Phase I/II trial of the safety and efficacy of shark cartilage in the treatment of advanced cancer," J. Clin. Oncol. 16 (1998): 3649–3655.

been approved by the FDA for the treatment of any cancers or disease, and there is disagreement over the findings within the scientific community. Research into AE-941 appears to have stalled.

To my knowledge, as of this writing, there has never been a trial conducted using powdered or liquid-form shark cartilage on newly diagnosed patients (not late-stage patients) who were not actively or previously treated using chemo, radiation, or other traditional therapies that might negate the efficacy or anti-angiogenesis effect of the cartilage.

Thus, it seems to me, at least, that there is hardly enough evidence to rule conclusively that shark cartilage is an ineffective cancer treatment, particularly in the way that my father and many others used it—without chemo and radiation, but alongside a healthful diet, bountiful self-care, mental-focus techniques like visualization, and with robust faith and prayer.

My father turned to self-treatment because there were no options or hopes for survival at the time of his diagnosis. The last twenty years, however, have shown incredible advancements in GBM treatment.

Encouragingly, there are more than three hundred active clinical trials targeting glioblastomas as of 2021, some of which have produced numerous glioblastoma super-survivors (i.e., patients who have survived more than a decade past their original diagnosis).

By far the most exciting and hopeful advancement in GBM research is the story of Sandra Hillburn.

Sandra Hillburn of Fort Lee, New Jersey, discovered a lemon-sized mass in her brain back in 2006. After a successful surgery, and completing a course of radiation, she was enrolled in a clinical trial at Duke University's Preston Robert Tisch Brain Tumor Center. The study of just over a dozen people tested a cancer vaccine therapy that targeted a protein called cytomegalovirus, or CMV, that is found in most glioblastoma brain tumors, but not in healthy brain tissue. Researchers extracted her white blood cells and exposed them to CMV. Hillburn then received a series of injections every six weeks for ten years at Duke that allowed her body to target the tumor cells using her own immune system. After ten years she received the injections about every six months, as her doctors felt her body had built up enough antibodies to fight tumor recurrence with less frequent treatment. Nearly sixteen years after her original diagnosis, Hillburn is leading a healthy and happy life, enjoying her nine grandchildren.

Sandy actually took a few minutes to speak to me for this book, and I must admit that reading her email to me and realizing that she was still alive after all this time left me in a puddle of happy tears. It was also funny because when I reached out to Duke University to ask whether Sandy was still alive, I was told something to the effect of, "Because of HIPPA we can't disclose if she's alive, but I'll give her your number and she can tell you yourself."

Sandy is a delightful, positive, and funny woman who is gracious and humble about her extraordinary story.

"I'm a very positive person," Sandy said. "My mother was the most positive person I knew, so it's hard not to be with a wonderful mother like her."

Sandy chalks her success up to her brilliantly talented surgeon who removed all of the tumor, to the incredibly talented and caring team at Duke University, and to the luck of the draw in the behavior of her tumor, which she described as more clearly defined than other GBMs.

"Everyone's story is different. I really just think I'm fortunate."

Sandy told me she also put in the extra legwork of altering her diet and upping her exercise. She walks several miles up steep hills every day. "Forget my head, it's my knees that are the problem now," she quipped.

Sandy had already spent years walking regularly with neighbors when she got her diagnosis at fifty-nine years old.

Sandy has also been following something called the Budwig Diet at the urging of her children. According to the Memorial Sloan Kettering Cancer Center, the Budwig Diet "consists of multiple daily servings of flaxseed oil and cottage cheese, as well as vegetables, fruits, and juices. Processed foods, meats, most dairy products, and sugar are prohibited."[9] It was developed by Dr. Johanna Budwig in the 1950s on the premise that the combination of foods would improve cellular functioning. Clinical studies have not been done on the Budwig Diet.

Sandy told me she went ten years without eating sugar until her youngest grandson introduced her to the guilty pleasure of mini ice cream cones. I think she's earned the teensy occasional treat.

She could not speak highly enough about the warmth and expert care she received from Duke University. "Anyone who is diagnosed with a glio should contact Duke," she said.

The codirector of the Duke Cancer Center Clinic, Dr. Henry Friedman, calls Sandy every weekend without fail. "He hasn't missed a weekend," Sandy said. "He was at a Duke University basketball game and he called me. He was at his son's wedding and he called me.

"I told him, 'I bet you didn't think I'd live this long, that you'd have to call and talk to me this long!' And he says, 'Yes I did! Yes I did!'"

Sandy is the longest and sole survivor of her small study. In interviews, the lead researcher and chief of neurosurgery at Duke, Dr. John Sampson, called Hillburn's results unprecedented, but he believes they have the data to prove that her case is more than just a fluke. He shied away from the word "cure" but said Hillburn was getting them as close to that definition as has ever been achieved.

[10]And Sandy isn't the only GBM super-survivor to have been treated at Duke University. David Fitting is one of, if not the longest living pediatric GBM survivor in America.

---

[9] Memorial Sloan Kettering Cancer Center, "Budwig Diet," 2020. Memorial Sloan Kettering Cancer Center, January 28, 2020. https://www.mskcc.org/cancer-care/integrative-medicine/herbs/budwig-diet-01.

[10] Lindsey Washburn, "Meet the Fort Lee woman who survived glioblastoma multiforme," NorthJersey.com, July 20, 2017. https://www.northjersey.com/story/news/health/2017/07/20/surviving-glioblastoma/495768001/.

David was a healthy ten-year-old boy when terrible headaches and prolonged episodes of déjà vu led to the discovery of a brain tumor. His family suffers from "Lynch Syndrome" which is a genetically elevated risk of cancer. After his first tumor was removed, he underwent a grueling course of chemo and radiation. The tumor returned exactly one year later and after his second surgery, David's parents were told that their son had just six weeks left to live.

That's when they reached out to Dr. Sridharan Gururangan at Duke and David began an experimental cocktail of chemotherapy drugs that had never been used for brain tumors before. He received an IV drop once a week for two years. Eighteen years later, he's alive and thriving, with just one cancer recurrence in his jaw (osteosarcoma) that was related to his exposure to radiation treatments as a child.

David is now working alongside the Glioblastoma Research Organization and shared his incredible story in *Newsweek*. "My experiences of cancer, especially the most recent one as an adult, have made me realize how strong I can be when I need to overcome adversity. When it matters, my default is positivity and optimism. Do I get down and upset, or lose my mind driving in Miami every day? Yes. But I know, when it really comes down to it, I'm a happy person who doesn't take life for granted."[11]

Another interesting point is that all of David's tumors were fully encapsulated, similar to Hillburn whose tumors were not as invasive as typical GBMs, and allowed for clean margins when removed.

It will be exciting to see if their incredible longevity can be recreated in other patients.

In 2019 the Henry Ford Center celebrated a decade of survival for a trio of GBM patients, Sasha Archer, Danielle Gillespie, and Chris Gee, after they enrolled in clinical trials there.

---

[11] David Fitting, "'I Was Diagnosed with Terminal Brain Cancer Twice as a Child—18 Years Later, I'm Still Alive,'" Newsweek, January 17, 2022. https://www.newsweek.com/terminal-brain-cancer-survivor-against-odds-1668722.

Henry Ford Center Director Dr. Steven Kalkanis said in a statement that while the average survival for glioblastomas is still under two years in the United States, and that even though less than one percent of patients live past eight years, "through innovative clinical trials and precision medicine, we've seen tripling of the number of very long-term survivors of the most malignant forms of brain cancer."[12]

Other research shows promise as well.

At Dana Farber Cancer Institute, the immunotherapy drug pembrolizumab in combination with radiation and multiple surgeries has allowed several GBM patients to blow by their original prognoses, with at least one patient living more than two years.[13]

Another clinical trial at Texas A&M was exploring promising immunotherapy. Published in *Clinical Cancer Research*, a journal of the American Association for Cancer Research, investigators tested a STING (Stimulator of Interferon Genes) drug injected directly into the glioblastoma of five dogs. The drug purports to stimulate the immune system to fight otherwise immunologically resistant cancer cells.

According to MRI scans taken throughout the ten-month trial, the drug induced a robust immune response in some of the dogs, some even after a single dose. That immune response reduced their tumor volume. One of the dogs had its tumor disappear completely. This could have very promising implications for human trials, which could begin soon. The researchers concluded that this therapy "can trigger a robust, innate anti-tumor immune

---

[12] Henry Ford Center, "Three Survivors of Glioblastoma Brain Cancer Celebrate 10 Years of Life Post-Diagnosis," Henry Ford Center, May 8, 2019. https://www.henryford.com/news/2019/05/three-survivors-of-glioblastoma-brain-cancer-celebrate-10-years-of-life

[13] Timothy F. Cloughesy et al., "Neoadjuvant Anti-PD-1 Immunotherapy Promotes a Survival Benefit with Intratumoral and Systemic Immune Responses in Recurrent Glioblastoma," Nature Medicine 25, no. 3 (2019): 477–86. https://doi.org/10.1038/s41591-018-0337-7.

response and may be highly effective on recalcitrant tumors such as glioblastoma."[14]

Immunotherapy has proved equally effective against other kinds of brain tumors. Former president Jimmy Carter suffered from a metastatic melanoma that traveled to his brain. This used to have similarly dire outcomes as glioblastomas, but immunotherapy drugs have dramatically improved the survival odds for melanoma.

Other therapies have been developed to lessen the toxic and damaging effects of standard treatments like radiation. Something called pulsed electromagnetic field therapy, or PEMF, is being used to help negate the necrosis and swelling caused by radiation, particularly in brain cancer patients, by promoting the regeneration of cells and boosting the immune system to weaken tumors.

Brain cancer survivor Nalie Agustin (@nalieagustin) has documented her battle and journey using PEMF. She shares that studies have found that "PEMF resulted in a significant reduction of blood flow to the tumor, with no changes in the rest of the brain. PEMF combined with chemotherapy leverages its effect by acting on tumor transmembrane permeability and consequently increasing drug concentration in tumor cells."[15]

At the same time, new research is demonstrating the full scope of just how damaging traditional treatments like chemotherapy can be.

A study out of Ohio State University published in the *International Journal of Molecular Sciences* set out to answer whether chemotherapy damages healthy cells to such an extent that it actually aids the spread of cancer cells. After treating mice with

---

[14] C. Elizabeth Boudreau et al., "Intratumoral Delivery of STING Agonist Results in Clinical Responses in Canine Glioblastoma," Clinical Cancer Research: An Official Journal of the American Association for Cancer Research 27, no. 20 (2021): 5528–35. https://doi.org/10.1158/1078-0432.CCR-21-1914.

[15] Nalie Agustin (@nalieagustin), "A metastasis to the brain was my biggest nightmare. We all know the prognosis is grim while treatments and therapeutic options are limited…" Instagram, December 16, 2020. https://www.instagram.com/p/CI3O34djDyi/.

chemo drugs, researchers observed that healthy blood vessels became "leaky," allowing for breast cancer cells to pass through, ultimately spreading and attaching to other parts of the body.

This is partly why my father was so strongly against chemotherapy in particular.

The research must continue.

Readers should note that my father's portion of this book addresses treatment options that were available at the time in the late '90s and early 2000s. I encourage everyone to do what my father did after his diagnosis and educate themselves as much as possible. Fight for every tidbit of information about treatment, trials, natural alternatives, and complementary therapies.

Because of the slow growth of my father's tumors, the three months my father was given to live turned into more than eight years. In that time, he had at least three additional successful surgeries to remove new tumors as they slowly grew. Ultimately, the tumors spread across his brain and body. He passed away in 2003, exactly eight years to the day that he took his first dose of shark cartilage. I was seventeen years old, sitting in a bookstore with my soon-to-be first boyfriend, Dwight, when I got the frantic call to come back home.

The Book

My father was diagnosed in 1995 and began writing this book in 1997, having already far outpaced his life expectancy. I have edited my father's book to correct his admittedly horrendous spelling and grammar. He was possibly dyslexic and very poor at writing, but he was relentless. I remember him typing away day after day, scouring the early internet for every scrap of information he could get his hands on. He set up meetings with authors, doctors, and nutritionists, tireless in his pursuit of information.

He wrote this book to give others hope.

Unfortunately, at the time of his death in 2003, none of us knew what to do with it.

Fifteen years later my mother rediscovered the book during a move and gave it to me. I remember holding that big, moldy, brown leather, zippered portfolio case and thumbing through the hundreds of still-intact pages inside and feeling myself fill with determination.

Now, as a journalist, and a parent myself, I was ready to ensure that my father's words did not die with him. His passion for life, his research, his courage, and his faith gave us many more years together as a family than we otherwise would have had. This book is his testimonial and my own, about the power of faith, of nutrition, nature, and of the power of the mind to overcome the obstacles before us. It is my mission now to get his words of hope out into the world where they belong.

Along with my father's story, at the end of this book you will find my investigation into the four factors I believe played the biggest roles in my father's longevity: Spirituality, Mental Fortitude, Nutrition, and Shark Cartilage.

You will also find an interview with international best-selling author and spiritualist Lorna Byrne, who talks to me about spiritual healing and finding peace at the end of one's life. I also speak with one of the living doctors who corresponded with my father, Dr. Eduardo A. Recio Roura of Spain. I share my fascinating and informative conversations with homeopathic oncologist Dr. Ian D. Bier, weight-loss champion Chuck Carroll, and best-selling author and motivational keynote speaker Michael Veltri.

I have provided a list of organizations and websites that may be helpful in your search for information at the end of this book. All of these resources and more, including my blog and ways to share this book, can be found at www.hopeforthehopeless book.com. You can also find the book on social media by searching @hopeforthehopelessbook.

While my father chose not to do chemo and radiation, this book is not a wholesale endorsement of that approach, merely a testimony of the life he lived. Many cancers respond very well to the latest mainstream therapies, and you should robustly research your options by consulting with your oncologists, nutritionists, specialists, and naturopathic cancer professionals to make the most sensible choice for you. My father forged his own way because there were no options and no hope for survival using traditional means of treatment at the time. This book does not claim to have discovered the cure for cancer or glioblastomas, but is an examination of my father's self-treatment.

I do not always know the perfect language to use to explain what my family experienced, but what I did witness is what drove me to journalism. The truth is always more compelling than fiction.

I share with you now my father's story as he wrote it.

1

Who Is Jimmy Blanco?

I was born in New Jersey, the first in my family to be born in the USA. My parents were Cuban immigrants who came from Cuba in 1955. We struggled through many tough years. As a baby, I slept in a drawer and was nearly eaten alive by rats. I was raised in Bayonne, New Jersey, and grew up in a rough neighborhood. Nothing has ever come easy for me. My father and mother were very hardworking.

When I was sixteen, my grades in school were slipping and I did not see high school preparing me for a good future. I was bright but restless, so when I turned seventeen I joined the army. I was promised a particular tech school but did not receive it. After my discharge, I joined the navy, and that did not work for me either. After that discharge, I went back to high school but did not graduate. I helped my dad with his flower shop. I always knew I had a higher purpose in life and was very frustrated because I did not know what it was.

I was smart but bored with regular school. I took my GED and passed with flying colors. I moved to Miami because I somehow felt that my destiny was there. When my dad sold his flower shop and moved to Miami, we both became taxi drivers. My father and I always worked together. I have always felt a strong bond and loyalty to him. I knew how much he sacrificed to raise me, my brothers, and my sister.

We worked a leased cab twenty-four hours a day. I worked

nights for twelve hours and my dad worked twelve hours in the day. We worked nonstop for eight months to save enough money to buy our own taxi medallion which allowed us to work as our own bosses. In 1982 I took on a second job working as a truck driver because the taxi business was slow, and that's where I met Elizabeth.

I delivered wines and Elizabeth was a secretary. I had fallen in love and planned to marry. I was twenty-four and I knew that it was time to start using the gifts God had given me. I started school for respiratory therapy. I knew I could do anything I put my mind to. I had a photographic memory and my strategy for being at the top of my class was to memorize whole chapters. I averaged high 90s throughout my courses. Soon I was married and became a registered respiratory therapist, registered pulmonary function technologist, and registered cardiovascular technologist with a blood gas license.

I obtained every degree possible in my field in less than five years. I worked in more than a dozen area hospitals because I wanted to learn how things were done in different hospitals. I was well known throughout Miami's respiratory circles. I thought I would make a difference, but after a few years, I realized I was not.

When ten years passed, I was mostly on cruise control. I didn't see myself accomplishing any of my goals. Then the miracle happened and my purpose in life was revealed to me. This was the higher purpose I knew I was born for. I was making a difference by beating incurable cancer and helping other cancer victims.

❧ 2 ❧

Miracle on 62nd Avenue

My story begins on October 26, 1995. I was unable to visit my mother on her birthday because of pure exhaustion. I had been feeling very tired for the past four months but shrugged it off as normal because of my hectic schedule of being a Little League manager for my son Jason's team and my crazy night-shift job.

I had pushed my body to its limit. I worked the night shift for twelve years, constantly adjusting my biological clock from being awake on nights then being awake on days when not working. This put a tremendous strain on my body, coupled with poor eating habits and the fact that I had always worked like an animal—two, three jobs at a time.

For about a year I had five jobs at one time, putting an average of twenty hours in each job. When I found a job that gave overtime, I did not need other jobs, but I put in an exaggerated number of hours. I would work sixteen- and twelve-hour shifts for thirty-five days in a row, then take a day off and work another fifty days. My peers were saying that I was not human, that I was an alien, and if you stabbed me I would not bleed.

I am a very focused person. When I put my mind to something, it gets accomplished. I have been described by my superiors as a person with the tenacity to get the job done. The doctors were complaining that I was making more money than they were. What they did not look at was the number of hours I had to work to make that kind of money. I have always been the kind of person that it was either all the way or nothing at all.

This craziness started when my wife and I looked at each other one day and said to each other, "What are we going to do?" We had two small babies, rented an apartment, and only had ten dollars to our name.

I thought to myself, *I am young and healthy with a new wife and kids. If I don't do something quickly, we are in big trouble.* So I worked and worked. My wife had another baby and we saved enough money to put a down payment on a house. When my last son, Jason, was three days old, we moved into the new house.

I asked my wife, Elizabeth, to stay home until the kids were at least five years old. A mother is so important to their children in the first five years. Elizabeth began to go to school for medical transcription and soon graduated and was able to work on a part-time basis. I have a medical family. My brother Tony is in radiology and worked his way up to manager of his department. My younger brother, Lazaro, is also in radiology with aspirations of being a doctor. My cousin Carlos is a surgical nurse, and now my wife is a medical transcriber, with myself being a respiratory therapist.

The hours I have worked in twelve years are equivalent to twenty-five years of the average person. I have worked with so many doctors, in so many hospitals. I have worked in so many intensive care units. I have worked with adults, pediatrics, and neonatal patients. My job was very stressful. I was maintaining very critical patients on life-support machines and participating in codes (CPR).

I must have witnessed at least a thousand adults, children, and babies die. Some due to trauma, others to disease, but whatever the reason it has been very stressful, especially when they are the same age as your own child.

It's not normal to see so many people die without it affecting you in one way or another. The frustration of being unable to help the majority of the patients was taking its toll on me. I thought to myself, *Why is it that in the most advanced country in the world, traditional therapies for illnesses such as cancer simply are not working?* Many days I could not wait to get home to hug my kids.

My wife thinks I am overprotective, and maybe I am, but she hasn't seen the things that I have. Over the years I've seen many doctors in action. I have worked with exceptional doctors. Some of them I consider the best in their field. I feel I have had the honor of working with some of the best surgeons, cardiologists, pulmonologists, nurses, and respiratory therapists anywhere.

What worries me is that I have also seen and worked with many that do not have a clue. They are the majority, and I have concluded that more than half the time they don't know what they are doing and are guessing. Maybe you have experienced taking your sick child to the doctor, and when your doctor cannot figure out what is wrong, he will always say it is a twenty-four-hour virus or it's a bug that's going around and everyone's getting it. Prevention is not taught or emphasized.

Doctors in this country are taught to treat the symptoms, not the underlying problem. If you have a headache, they'll tell you to take acetaminophen. If you have a fever, headache, or any other symptom, it means that your body is trying to tell you that there is something wrong. What the doctors do too often is mask the problem, probably unintentionally, by treating the symptoms. Before you know it, your illness may have progressed too far, then it's too late.

I was really fed up with the profession I chose, and many times I tried to change it. I bought a racehorse, raising and training him from six months old. After two years of hard work and more overtime to be able to pay for his training at Hialeah and Calder Racetracks, it was all for nothing. Three days before his first race I received a phone call from the track that told me they were putting my horse down due to a broken leg suffered during training. It was a devastating blow to me and a shattered dream I had had since childhood. It was also a tremendous financial blow because I did not have him insured.

I loved horses all of my life, and this was my way out of the medical field and to do something I loved. I do not know why things happened the way they did, but I comforted my wife by telling her that things happened for the best.

There is a blessing in every problem; you just have to put your faith in God and ask Him to guide you. A few years later I tried to open a wholesale business, and it failed miserably. I tried a 1-900 business and did not make a penny. When I invested in gold, it dropped and I lost money again. There was no escaping it. For some reason, I was meant to stay where I was and bear witness to all the hardship, suffering, and dying until God said it was enough.

In February of 1995, I began to cut back on my hours to relieve some stress and spend more time with my three children. I began managing my six-year-old son's baseball team and I also coached on my eight-year-old's team. This relieved a lot of stress in the beginning, but when I was caught up in a race for first place, my competitive personality emerged, and it added to my stress.

Between my work and a pennant race, I was killing myself. Coupled this with my diet of fast foods for a fast life and I was reaching my physical limitation without even knowing it.

I knew something was wrong with me. I just did not know what. I began to ask for a vacation and was repeatedly denied due to a staffing shortage. I was constantly fatigued, with numbness in my left hand in the morning upon arising. I ignored the symptoms and rationalized it was due to dead nerves on my left wrist because of surgery I had twenty-two years previous when I was fifteen. It must be getting worse because of my age, or maybe I was sleeping on it.

I was stumbling over my feet at work and people were laughing at me. "It must be because I'm tired," I rationalized. Working in the medical field for so long and working with neurological patients all the time, I should have figured out something was very wrong and I needed to have it checked.

No one ever thinks that something will happen to them, and I was no different. I would say to myself, *I am only thirty-seven years old and have never been sick a day in my life.* My lack of confidence in doctors is what stopped me from checking out my symptoms.

On October 26, 1995, it was my mother's birthday, and I was unable to see her because I was in bed the whole day. I was barely able to get up for work, and my wife had a hard time trying to wake me up at 10:30 p.m. She wanted me to call out sick, and so did my nine-year-old daughter, who was crying and telling me to stay because she thought that something bad was going to happen. I knew I could not, because they had been giving people a hard time over staffing shortage.

I had lent my car to my dad, so I was going to take my scooter as I have done many times before, but Elizabeth insisted I take our new van.

The route I always take is through the expressway, then when I'm close to the hospital I go by way of residential streets. As I approached the hospital, I looked at my watch to see if I was going to be on time. It was 10:50 p.m., so I was going to make it. Or so I thought. I was only a few blocks away. All of a sudden my left hand began to shake, followed by the rest of my body. I immediately became blind and deaf. After a few seconds, I began to realize what was happening thanks to my twelve years in the medical field. I was having a grand mal seizure.

The last thing I remember seeing was two oncoming cars. I was on Sixty-Second Avenue, a small two-lane road. I thought to myself, *I have to take my foot off the accelerator and I have to try to place my right hand on the wheel.* Of course, I had no control to do either. I was hoping that the van would go to the right instead of the left, where I would surely crash head-on into the approaching traffic. I was unconscious within five seconds.

I awoke to some tapping on my window, and to my amazement I was alive. It was a miracle of God that I was not killed in the accident. God had taken control of the wheel and led me to a soft crash in front of a house just one block from my work. I did not have a scratch on me; the only damage to my car was a reflector in the front.

A year later I found out the lady that lives in the house where I crashed had a custom of checking in front of her house before she goes to bed. She spotted me and her son called fire rescue. If I had crashed in front of another house, I may have been there all night. This may have been fatal.

My first thoughts when I revived were angry. I was angry at myself. *What have I done now?* People were staring at me from the house. I looked at my watch; it was midnight. "I can't believe that I'm late," I said to myself. I was very lethargic. My next thoughts were that I was at home still sleeping and this was all a nightmare. Reality set in when I saw three police officers tapping at my window again. I knew what they were thinking—they thought I was a drunk driver.

Unfortunately, living in Miami, that is not an uncommon scenario for them. I lowered the window with my head still weaving back and forth and asked the officer, "May I help you?" Now I looked like I was on drugs or something.

He asked me to step out of the vehicle, which I proceeded to do, stumbling all over the place. Then he wanted my driver's license, and I had to go back into the van, just barely making it out with my license. A paramedic was looking at my eyes very closely, and I remember him telling another officer that this was a medical problem.

I was immediately placed in the ambulance and transported to the nearest adult hospital. As I rode in the ambulance, I thought of my wife and how she would react to the dreaded phone call— that dreadful phone call no one ever wants to receive, telling her that a loved one has been in an accident and is in the emergency room.

The paramedic asked me a lot of questions that I don't remember because my mind was somewhere else. When I arrived at the emergency room, I was moved from the stretcher to the bed. The paramedic and the nurse looked at each other when they saw that as a result of the grand mal seizure, I had lost all control of my bodily functions. One of the nurses asked if I wanted to call anyone, and I had her call my work, who was still awaiting my arrival. I also had them call my wife. When there was no answer, I had them call my parents' house. They put in a heparin lock and drew all the blood they needed.

I was still delirious, and I remember them asking more questions about my medical history. I told them that I've been very healthy all my life and I didn't even have a doctor. The first people I saw were my dad and mom. I was very happy to see them. My dad was strong, always reassuring, telling me everything was all right. I knew my mom was very scared; she was telling the nurses that I was a very good boy. This is typical of most moms who love their children. I saw and heard the fear and anguish in her voice and eyes as she stroked my arms up and down. My mom had good reason to be afraid.

I knew that a seizure was an indication of brain dysfunction, most probably a tumor of some kind. I should have been afraid, too, but I was too tired to be concerned. They took me for a CAT scan, and when the doctor came in to tell me I had a seven-centimeter tumor in my right frontal hemisphere, I was not surprised.

At this point, my wife arrived and my parents were outside the ER crying. I was always joking with my wife that I was going to die or retire before the age of forty. The first thing I told her was, "I told you so." I didn't want her to be worried about me, especially since she now had the extra duty of taking care of the three kids on her own.

"I'm always right and you never listen to me," I told her.

"You didn't have to be right about this!" she replied. I was trying very hard to keep good humor about the whole thing. The doctors said they had to do an MRI to confirm and get a better picture of what it was.

I am extremely claustrophobic, and I thought I was going to have problems in this coffin-type procedure. I didn't, because I was totally out of it. The MRI confirmed the seriousness of the situation. The neurologist on call came in to see me. He explained to me that this was a life-threatening situation and I needed emergency surgery. I did not know the neurologist, but he seemed very good.

I always had a lot of respect for surgeons. In a life-threatening situation, they are excellent. I've seen them work miracles. The tumor had invaded most of the right side of my brain and was already deviating two centimeters past the midline into the left side of my brain.

I began searching deep inside and talking to God to see why I had found myself in this situation. I remembered six months previous I had gone to the beach to have a one-on-one conversation with God. I prayed that He would please get me out of the profession I was in because I wasn't helping anyone. I couldn't stand to see children suffering and dying anymore.

That's when I realized that my prayers were answered and everything was going to be all right, because I was in God's hands now. One must be careful of what they pray for; they just might get it. Prayers are not always answered as one expects. Who are we to say how God should do things? Right away I knew that He would turn this whole problem into a blessing. I believe that illness comes from the devil. I also believe that God allowed the devil to do his evil deed on me because He would turn it into a blessing.

I was transported up to the intensive care unit, where they needed to stabilize me first. I was treated extremely well in this hospital. The ICU nurses were very nice and helpful.

I really liked the hospital, but I wanted to be transferred to another hospital for the surgery. The reason was that I had worked there for four years and I knew all the nurses, therapists, and intensive care staff. I was transported to that hospital and my surgery was scheduled for Halloween 1995, of all days. Halloween has not been very good for me. Well, I didn't worry about Devil's Day, because I knew the Lord would be with me. I was put in a regular room in the neurologic wing. Many of my friends and family came to visit.

I wasn't much of a host, because I knew what lay ahead for me was going to be very tough. Finally, the day came and the neurological surgeon came to talk to me about the procedure and answer my questions.

I told him that my main worry about the surgery was leaving a piece of my skull out. I wanted either my own skull back or a plate, but did not want to leave my brain unprotected. I've seen many craniotomies on neurological patients and they are left with this massive sunk-in hole in their heads. That is totally unacceptable. He told me he would put my own skull back. I guess there have been advances in this area from what I have seen.

My other worry was that they might leave me awake for the surgery. I've seen brain surgery where the patients are awake so that the doctors can communicate with the patient. This assists the surgeon so they do not cut in the wrong area. I had flashbacks of the times that I was a respiratory therapy instructor and I would take my students to the hospital's medical examiner's department to see autopsies being performed. One of the most gruesome sights to see was when they would drill a cadaver's head open and remove the brain.

He reassured me that they'd use general anesthesia. I wasn't too worried about that, even though I should have been. I've seen patients that died because either the anesthesiologists made an error or the patient was allergic to the general anesthesia and died. There is also the possibility that the doctor makes a mistake or I get an infection of some kind. I believe the more you know, the more you have to worry about. Then again, whether you know or you don't, the problems still exist, so it's better to know and be prepared for what's ahead.

As I was wheeled through the hallways to the surgery preparation room on the stretcher, I stared up into the lights. I was remembering the many times I was on the other end, wheeling someone else to surgery or the intensive care or CAT scan and MRI. I focused my attention on the people who were providing my care and wondered if I was as caring as I should have been when I was in their place.

I remembered that sometimes I was and other times I wasn't. I also understood that healthcare professionals get more desensitized as the years pile on. It's a defensive mechanism many people use to protect themselves from going crazy. No one likes to get too emotionally involved with their patients, because many do not make it. One hopes it never happens to them.

I remembered the very first cardiac arrest that I witnessed. I was just a student at a local hospital. I was not allowed to participate, just observe. I was in the intensive care unit when they called a code blue (cardiac arrest). Everyone sprang into action. The respiratory therapist began to pump on his chest, assisted the doctor in intubating the patient, and they took their blood gas. The nurses started their IVs and proceeded to give the patient the lifesaving medications needed to bring him back to life.

The doctor was giving orders of what medications were needed. "Prepare the paddle to shock the heart, more lidocaine," etc. It all looked very professional, but something was missing.

There was no human compassion for this poor man. His wife was at the door of the unit crying her eyes out. Everyone in the code, from doctors to therapists to nurses, were talking about this like it was a social event. They were cracking jokes, talking about what they were going to do on the weekend and what they'd done the other day.

I was in a state of shock! I couldn't believe what I was witnessing. I asked myself, *Is this the field that I have chosen for a career?* Eventually, the patient died and they stopped trying to bring him back. Not one of them stopped to look back to see how degrading they left this poor man. He looked like a mess, with the endotracheal tube still hanging out of his mouth, his chest hairs burnt from the electric paddle with the stench burning flesh, his arms hanging over the sides, his eyes opened with needles and gauze all over him. Blood everywhere, it was a disaster.

I looked up into a corner and I knew this man was looking

down at himself. I wonder what he must have thought of the insensitive people that were caring for him. I felt I was communicating with this man I've never known. I was apologizing to him and asking the Lord to take him into His arms.

Meanwhile, everyone had gone back into the staff lounge, still joking, and returned to eating as if nothing had happened. The wife was crying hysterically and no one comforted her. It was a terrible first impression of the medical field. Later I would discover that this was the norm and not the exception.

So when I arrived in the preparation room a very nice nurse inserted a sixteen-gauge needle into my right wrist for the anesthesia. "Excellent job," I told her. They allowed me to speak briefly with my family. I didn't expect to come out of surgery alive, so I told my parents that I loved them. I hugged my wife, Elizabeth, and whispered in her ear that I loved her. This was a very emotional moment for me because I hardly ever told Elizabeth that I loved her, but she always knew that I did.

I prayed to God that He wouldn't leave my three children fatherless. In case I didn't make it, at least they would know that I loved them. I've never been the kind of guy that expresses my emotions with words. Words are cheap and anyone can say "I love you." I always expressed my love by the actions I did for people and family.

The surgeon came in to see me and that was the last thing I remembered, because they had slipped something in my IV line without me seeing. The next thing I remembered was waking up in the recovery room. I was amazed again that God had blessed me with another miracle and got me through a major surgery such as this. I was very delirious from the anesthesia still and I don't remember much. I do vaguely remember my dad coming in. I was so happy to see him that I tried to get up to put my arms around him. They told him to leave. I later heard it was because they didn't want to excite me.

I was taken to the intensive care unit, where I knew I would be in good hands. I've worked with many of these nurses and knew them to be amongst the finest in Miami-Dade County. I was in excruciating pain and my head was wrapped like a mummy. The first nurse I had was Cathy; I remembered her as being excellent and very caring.

One of the first things I felt I needed was a desperate back rub. I didn't even have to ask for it. Cathy took it upon herself to do it. It is absolutely incredible how such a little gesture to a sick patient can bring so much relief. Most healthcare providers don't even realize this until they themselves are on the other side. I know I definitely learned something that day.

They had amazing patience with all the calls and family and friends that were trying to see me and get information. I was running a high fever and I was given lots of pain medication. The first three faces I saw entering my room were three coworkers. They were Diana, George, and Marline.

They knew how to get around and they sneaked in. I was in shock because they were three people from a different shift who I thought disliked me. Life is full of lessons, and at that moment I learned that a person's true character emerges during hard times. The coworkers I thought were my closest friends weren't there, yet these three who I barely even spoke to were there. I was happy to see them and thanked them for being concerned enough to come to see me.

I had the room very dark because the lights bothered me. During the time I was asleep, I would wake up occasionally, and I saw a dark figure walking around the room. I couldn't quite figure out who it was, but I would hear him talking to himself. He appeared very concerned. It turned out to be Michael, my brother-in-law, whom I had not even met yet. I thought that was very thoughtful of him.

The next two nurses that took care of me were Ivone and Isabell. They were both excellent.

On the next day, the neurosurgeon removed my bandages and said I was to go to the floors. I begged him to leave me one more day because I didn't feel I was ready to go to the floors, where I knew that the nurses are swamped with patients and the care wouldn't be as good.

My pleas fell on deaf ears and I was transferred to the floors. I spent a lot of time sleeping and resting. I had some wonderful nurses named Maria and Robin during the day, but terrible nurses at night. That's why my wonderful dad, bless his soul, would stay with me at night even though he was sick himself.

I liked my neurosurgeon and I think he did an excellent job of saving my life. For that, I thank him from the bottom of my heart. I wasn't recovering as fast as the neurologist wanted me to. He wanted me to recover from major brain surgery in three days and ship me home as soon as he could. The only problem was that I knew the game he was playing. He forgot that I've been in the medical field for twelve years.

He would come in the morning and open all my shades and let the light in, waking me up from a sound sleep. I understand that he wanted to see me more active, but some people take longer than others to recover.

"It looks like you could go home," he said.

I said, "Listen, Doc, I can barely move, I need help to go to the bathroom, I have staples in my head, I have a tremendous head-ache, I'm twitching all day, and I'm not going anywhere until I'm better."

I know that hospitals and doctors are paid by the diagnosis, meaning they get a certain amount of money for my brain tumor, and if they could get the patient out sooner with the least number of tests possible, then the doctor and the hospital benefit from all the extra cash.

If it takes the patient longer to recover than the allotted time and money given by the insurance companies, then the hospitals and doctors lose money. Now we all know that hospitals have no intention of losing money—after all, this is a business. I'm not say-ing that this is what was happening here, but it seemed so at the time.

A hospital RN from oncology had come to talk to me before.

"If there is anything I can do for you, please call me. I'm here to help you." After the doctor talked to me, I called her for help.

"What are they doing for you here that they can't do for you at home?" she asked. This question made me very angry and upset. I told her that in the hospital they were giving me my medications on time, I was continually monitored for my twitching, they were doing blood tests in the mornings to check my anti-seizure medication level, and I was getting the rest I needed to recover. None of these things could be done at home, especially since my wife works and my three young children would not let me rest. I told her I wasn't going anywhere until I was ambulatory.

The next day the doctor came in and said, "Maybe it's a good idea to leave you here for three more days. That way we could remove those staples from your head and you could meet your oncologist." He had a totally different attitude. The reason being is they don't want trouble with patients that know their rights.

"Okay, Doc, where do we go from here?" my dad asked.

"We have to start a very aggressive treatment of chemotherapy and radiation. Time is of the essence."

"How long did this tumor take to grow to seven centimeters?" I asked.

"It grew in about three months," he replied.

"What causes brain tumors, and did the cellular phone I recently began using have anything to do with it?"

"We don't know," he replied. He told me I had three to six months to live. I was too upset to ask any more questions, so I made an appointment to see him.

I was taken to the cancer ward to prepare for radiation treatments. I asked questions on side effects, and there were so many that it just depressed me even more. They set me up for a week of simulations and preparations to start radiation the following week. Meanwhile, I went to see my self-appointed oncologist to ask more questions. I brought my brother Tony and my wife, Elizabeth, along to make sure I understood everything correctly.

His big thing was chemotherapy. "You want me to take chemotherapy, but could you explain to me how this drug"—I wanted to say poison—"is going to cross the blood-brain barrier? Won't it destroy my immune system along with my healthy organs?"

"The new drugs do cross the blood-brain barrier, and it will destroy the bad cells," he responded.

"Won't it destroy the good cells along with the bad?" I asked.

"Yes, but you need to weigh your options."

"Could I speak to someone who has what I have and is taking chemotherapy so I could ask them questions?"

His response was, "No!"

"Why, are they all dead?" I asked.

"Yes," was his answer.

His answer and the cold stare in his eyes were so unbelievable to me. Aren't doctors there to give one hope? I could not help but laugh; it sounded like the punchline a standup comedian would make. I already had my doubts that he had my well-being in mind. His office appeared like a drive-through chemo station. He spoke very fast, as if he had minimal time to spend on you. Time is money, and I had very good insurance with a limit of one million dollars.

I wonder if that is the reason he was pushing chemotherapy on me so much, especially knowing that it would not help in my case. Through his admission, he couldn't refer me to any patient with a brain tumor that had survived the chemotherapy. I wondered what really killed those patients—the tumor, or the destruction of the immune system with the chemotherapy.

I asked him, "Wouldn't the chemotherapy adversely affect my other vital organs with no guarantee of reaching the brain?"

"Yes, there's a strong possibility, but you're young."

What I rationalized from that answer was that he didn't believe I was going to live long enough to worry about my other organs.

"So why would I do that to myself? Is chemotherapy going to cure me?"

"No, there is no cure for what you have. It will allow you

to live about twenty more weeks than you would if you don't take it."

This was the easiest decision I've ever had to make. At that moment I remembered the scene in the waiting room where I saw one of his patients waiting for her chemotherapy and eating a big, giant quarter-pounder with cheese.

I told myself, *There are cancer patients who are not even given instructions on proper nutrition.* That convinced me that this doctor was not interested in whether I recovered. He was a very nice man and gave me prescriptions for anything I asked for. He appeared to be a caring man. I do not like to judge people. I don't know if he's out for the buck or if he just doesn't know that chemotherapy is poison. It's not logical to me that one could expect to heal a patient who is suffering from cancer, with their immune system compromised already, to get better by poisoning them with chemotherapy.

Now the body not only has to fight cancer but also the poison. With a weakened immune system to begin with, it's no wonder patients get so sick while taking this stuff. Compounding the problem, they don't emphasize changing their diet or proper nutrition. I made my decision to not take chemotherapy.

The next decision was radiation. Should I, or shouldn't I?

What came to mind when contemplating this decision was all those cancer patients I've treated throughout the years. I've seen them suffering from the terrible side effects of radiation and chemotherapy. At work, what bothered me the most was when I would be assigned to the cancer ward. The small children staring up at you with those beautiful eyes hoping that you could relieve their pain. I would get too emotional and would do anything in my power not to be assigned there.

There is one particular girl I remember who was in the same elementary school as my children. I came to hear about her at a school festival. All the children were having a great time. One of the school workers asked me to bring my kids to sign a giant get-well card. This card was going to be sent to one of the kids that was sick with cancer (lymphoma). She was doing chemotherapy.

I asked her what room she was in, because I worked at the hospital and would like to go see her. My day was ruined by that news. I saw all those healthy children playing and couldn't help but think it could be anyone's child.

I began to videotape the event with the idea of making a copy and giving it to her in the hospital so she wouldn't feel like she missed all the fun. My daughter Jamie won a cake in the game of musical chairs, and I asked her if she would like to donate it to the little sick girl in the hospital. She said yes.

That night while at work, I went to see this little girl I didn't know. When I walked into that room I saw this gorgeous five-year-old girl. She was suffering so much from the side effects of chemotherapy. I had to fight back my tears. I couldn't believe that with the billions of dollars we have spent in this country over the years on research, we are no closer now than we were twenty or thirty years ago to find the cure or the causes of most, if not all, cancers. We don't know how to prevent or cure it without destroying other vital organs.

Chemotherapy and radiation are like taking your car to the mechanic to get fixed. They fix one thing and break something else so that you'll have to come back and give them more business. Where is all that taxpayer money going? Do they really want to find a cure? Are they afraid that their research money will stop coming in if they do? Do the pharmaceutical companies want Americans sick so they can profit from drug sales? I don't know the answers to these questions, but I do know that funds would be more wisely used on research for alternative therapies that show promise, like shark cartilage. As I stood there watching this child, I asked God, "Why? Why such an innocent child?"

I was so emotional. Instinctively I asked God, "Take me instead, Lord."

As soon as I said that, I said to myself, "What am I saying? I have three small kids of my own that need their father."

I couldn't work that night without thinking of her. Later I learned never to ask God why. I made the mistake that most healthcare professionals avoid at all costs. That is to get emotionally involved with a patient. You set yourself up for a big disappointment if they don't make it.

I decided to refuse all conventional treatment, including chemotherapy and radiation. If God wanted me to die in three months, I would, and if He did not, I would not. I figured if God really wanted me to die, I would have crashed head on with those oncoming cars. I was spared for a reason. I didn't know the reason, but now, it appears to me it was to bring hope to others like me.

When I returned home, I tried my best to appear strong for my children. I was trying to shelter them from the truth. People advised me to tell them that I was dying. I refused. How do you tell a six-, eight-, and nine-year-old that their daddy has cancer and, according to the doctors, is going to die in three months?

They did not understand what was happening to me. They acted as if nothing happened. I was advised to tell the children before they heard it from someone else so they would be prepared and better able to cope with my death. I was constantly telling them to be quiet, and my patience was all but exhausted.

After leaving the hospital, any little sound was amplified a thousand times in my head. One day they were making a lot of noise and giving me a terrible headache. I asked them all to sit down so that I could explain to them why their father was so irritable when they would play and make so much noise.

I pleaded with them to understand that just because I was out of the hospital did not mean that I was well. "Your dad is very, very sick. You can't see it because what is making me sick is inside my head." I was very emotional and began to cry. "You must help me get well by behaving and not making noise, because that hurts me very much. The doctor says I have cancer and only have a little time to live."

At this point, I was so angry with myself. Angry because I was not going to be there for my children. I felt sorrow for them that they would have to grow up with no father to guide them in the years that followed. Who would be there for them when they had problems in school or when they needed fatherly advice when it came to morals, dating, jobs, career, etc.? Who would play ball with them and care for them the way I had? Who would protect them and my wife? I had hundreds of questions flash in my head and I was mad. I asked them all to hug me as I cried.

After that day, I think they began to understand the seriousness of the situation. They never saw their daddy cry, so they knew it was serious. As time passed and the months came and went, they began to have faith and confidence that their father was going to beat this dreaded disease. I asked them to grow up that day. That made me feel even more guilty. Guilty of robbing them of their innocence and their childhood, forcing them to understand something that they were too young to understand. Guilty for bringing trauma into their lives.

❧ 3 ❧

The Fourth Opinion

I felt that if I was going to write a book and make any claims of success, I should go to extraordinary lengths to prove that my diagnosis of a deadly glioblastoma multiforme was correct. I had my tissue diagnosed at the hospital where I had my surgery. My tissue was sent to another major northeastern hospital for a second opinion, with the same results. I then requested a slide of my tissue and took it to another independent pathologist for a third opinion. He came back with the same results. I was not satisfied. I still had my doubts.

How could I know that this tissue that had been diagnosed with a glioblastoma multiforme grade IV was really my tissue? This was a tough question. I searched for a way to answer for the next eleven months with no success. Everyone assured me that there was no way there could have been a mistake, because I was most probably the only brain tumor surgery in the whole hospital that day, or week for that matter. Brain surgery is very rare. The reason I could not rest until I knew the truth was that others with my diagnosis weren't doing as well as I was.

They either died or had multiple surgeries due to the speed at which these tumors grow. I concluded that there were only two possible scenarios: One, this tissue was not mine and I was misdiagnosed. Or two, the alternative treatment I chose, which included the shark cartilage, was really working. Maybe the fact that I never subjected my body to the poisons of chemo-therapy and radiation was beneficial also.

Whichever the truth was, I was in good shape compared to others. If it wasn't my tissue, then there was a good chance my tumor was less deadly than first thought. If it was my tissue, then I was living proof that radiation and chemotherapy are not necessary for my type of tumor. Also, it may prove that the shark cartilage with the supplements could bring hope for future patients with brain tumors.

A breakthrough in my search came when I spoke to someone from my church who gave me the name of a company. I con-tacted them and they weren't able to help, but they forwarded my name to someone that could. They worked in forensics and normally worked on paternity cases, matching children to their biological parents. My request was out of the ordinary, but nevertheless they could match my tissue to some cheek cells or blood sample that I would provide.

I had a paraffin block of my tumor that was given to me by the hospital cut to as close to one micron as possible. At my own expense, I sent out ten slides along with my cheek swab. This test would verify if this indeed was my tissue or not. After three weeks of anticipation, the results weren't coming in.

I couldn't wait any longer; I just had to call them. "How is the test going?" I asked.

"We've done only three of ten tests so far, but the results are coming in pretty consistent with your DNA profile. These tests are not conclusive, and we must wait until all the tests are com-plete to know for sure."

A week and a half later, I called again. After speaking to the forensics lab for the second time, reality finally began to set in.

"We've done nine tests and it appears to be consistent with your profile. The odds are one in millions that it's not yours."

I was a little depressed after speaking to them, because a part of me was hoping that this was all some kind of a mix-up or something. After receiving the news, I spent some time reflecting on what this all meant. I came to the conclusion that this was the final proof that indeed God has worked a miracle on me. The shark cartilage was a Godsend.

I don't know why God has spared me. Maybe it was so that I could write this book and make others who are suffering from this disease aware of a possible treatment. Maybe it's to bring hope to the hopeless. Maybe it's to open the eyes of the doctors. Maybe it's to open the eyes to the public about the medical establishment's submissive attitude toward finding an alternative method of treating brain cancer. Maybe it is for some other reason that I am not aware of. Whatever the reason, I just pray every day that God guides me in the direction He wishes me to go. I pray that He gives me the strength to do His will.

A few weeks later, I received the final word.

"Yes, the tissues match."

The odds that this was not my tissue were fifty-two million to one.

The last question to myself was, maybe this new block of tissue that I had analyzed for DNA was indeed mine, but was it a glioblastoma multiforme? I never had it diagnosed before sending it for DNA analysis. I was really reaching for straws, but just maybe it wasn't a glioblastoma. I took the samples that I received back from the test to have it diagnosed again to see if this new block was also glioblastoma multiforme grade IV. The results were identical to the previous four opinions. Now, I finally had to accept the facts. I wish the medical doctors would also accept the facts. The facts are, yes, I had a glioblastoma multiforme grade IV. No, I did not take the standard treatment of radiation and chemotherapy. Yes, there is hope for patients with this diagnosis, if they wouldn't be so closed-minded. In battling cancer, yes, shark cartilage works if administered properly with the proper brand and dosages.

Contributing factors that are not acknowledged as beneficial:

1. Faith and prayers for yourself and by others
2. A positive state of mind
3. Remaining stress-free
4. Shark cartilage
5. Herbs and supplements
6. Meditation, visualization, and hypnosis
7. Diet and nutrition

4

Radiation Option

I didn't know much about radiation. I only knew that there is radiation in atomic bombs and it killed a lot of people in Japan to end World War II. I also knew that all x-ray technicians wear a special badge to monitor how much radiation they are exposed to and are not to receive more than a certain amount. I went to see the doctor who was to do my radiation treatments. He seemed to be a nice guy and caring. I had to sign a lot of papers saying that I was aware of all the possible side effects. They were very depressing.

It looked as though it was written by a hospital lawyer; everything, including the kitchen sink, was thrown into the document. The possible side effects include headaches, hair loss, low blood counts, skin redness, itching, fatigue. Possible complications include damage to the brain, skin, hair loss, damage to vision or sight, even severe enough to cause death.

The risk of side effects or complications and their severity may be increased because of prior or subsequent chemotherapy or surgery. I was hoping to get some hope from him on my prognosis, but all he did was confirm what every other doctor had already said—that there is no hope of recovery.

They began a few days of what they call radiation simulations. The technician prepared me on a table and took a series of x-rays. He also made a special mask that conformed to my facial features. On my next visit, the technician put the mask on and took more x-rays, and blasted me with some laser beams. The mask was very tight, and I wasn't allowed to move. It was very scary for me, and I was in the medical field. I could only imagine how the average person must feel.

Radiation may be good for some types of cancer, but for my type it was not worth the effort. You may be subjecting yourself to complications that you did not have before. I have not seen it work on anyone who has a glioblastoma, and I have spoken with quite a few. I don't agree with the theory that it buys you time.

I've seen people react differently to radiation. In some people, it retarded the growth of the tumor temporarily, only to have it start growing again after the treatment stopped. While for others, I've heard that it made it spread to other locations of the brain and even made it grow faster. Personally, I believe the benefits do not outweigh the risks of the side effects.

Most importantly, note that radiation is not a cure. Your body can only tolerate a certain amount of radiation, so one can only take the treatment so often and that's it. After that, radiation is not an option any longer. If it doesn't cure you, then you are accomplishing only two things by doing the procedure: First, you are subjecting your body to a poison that may cause you other problems. Second, you are lining the pockets of the already rich cancer centers and doctors. I've been told that I should have done conventional treatment first, before doing alternatives.

I respond by saying, why would I do a treatment *proven ineffective* for my kind of cancer? Radiation has been proven not to prevent glioblastoma multiforme from eventually regrowing. It is also proven that it is not a cure. Chemotherapy is not even worth mentioning.

❦ 5 ❧

Fight for What's Yours

After my simulation, I went to the hospital to get my medical records. This is something all patients should do. One must take control of their own health and not just listen to what their doctors tell them, no matter how nice or how long they've known them. Doctors can be wrong; they are just human like the rest of us. Many doctors like to play God, but the bottom line is you want to get as many opinions as possible and make a consensus of their recommendations. That is why you need your medical records, to facilitate this process.

You might have a hard time getting them if you don't know your rights. Make sure you ask for *all* your records from the moment of admission. They usually will make you sign a paper and wait three days. When I went back in three days, they only gave me ten sheets of paper. I asked them, "What's this?"

They said, "This is all your pertinent information."

I asked, "Says who? Who are you to say what's pertinent and what's not? As far as I'm concerned, every sheet of paper in my chart is pertinent." I wanted my nurses' notes, my doctors' progress notes, my lab results, etc. I had just come out of the hospital, was very weak, and not in any condition to argue or get upset, yet I was forced to by insensitive employees.

The next story they gave me was, "Well, it's going to cost you a dollar a sheet, and there are about two hundred sheets." My blood was boiling.

"I'm not paying you one red cent, because every piece of paper you have with my name on it is my property."

Whenever you need something from a department in a hospital, always ask to speak to the manager of the department. Cut out all the workers and supervisors for best results.

My brother Tony spoke to the department head, and the next day I had all my records with no problems. Another time I had to get more records I had to go through the same baloney. I told the guy that I was not in the mood for the runaround, and he told me to just write down that it was for the doctor and not for me.

I told him, "I'll write whatever you want, but I'm taking my records."

The reason they make it so difficult for you to obtain your records is that they don't want you to find out too much about what they did to you during your admission. If they charged you for a procedure that wasn't done or wasn't ordered by a doctor for whatever reason, even if the doctor forgot to write the order and it was done, you are not responsible for that bill.

They are also afraid of lawsuits. You might find out that a nurse messed up by giving you the wrong medication or they did an unnecessary procedure or a therapist documented a procedure that was never done. You would never know unless you had the records and compared the procedures ordered with what you were billed for.

My next stop was radiology. I needed to pick up my MRI, x-rays, and CAT scan. Here I didn't have much trouble. Make sure you know exactly what you had done, because they'll only give you what you ask for, even though you might have something else there. Also, ask for the originals, not copies.

My next stop was the pathology department. This was my worst stop. I was given the cold shoulder and runaround treatment. I simply wanted the slides with my brain tissue on them. I spoke to the supervisor and asked her if I could speak to the pathologist that examined my tumor and diagnosed me with this terminal incurable disease.

Her answer was, "No, what for? Why do you want your brain tissue?"

"Well, for one thing, it's mine, and I would like to have it analyzed for a second opinion," I said to her.

She said, "We already sent it for a second opinion."

"Well, can I have the telephone number there so I could call in reference to my pathology?"

She was very reluctant with a poor attitude, giving me dirty looks, and I didn't have any more energy to continue arguing. I know that the brain tissue is mine and I'd get it later, even if it meant getting a lawyer. When I finally got home, I was so disgusted with the way hospitals are run that I felt like writing a letter to my congressman. Instead, I went to sleep. I knew that would have been a waste of my time and energy. Months later, I emailed many congressmen and senators. I never received a response from any of them.

You must be your own best advocate.

6

The Gamma Knife Option

G amma knife was something new to me. I heard it was a very good option for me and I was excited to check it out. The gamma knife is focused radiation on a tumor. The tumor must be of a certain size, no larger than a couple of centimeters, I believe. It sounded great, so I made an appointment to see one of the leading physicians working with the gamma knife. I discovered that if it sounds too good to be true, it is too good to be true.

Radiation is radiation, no matter how you slice it. When you want to try some new form of treatment, you should ask to speak to former patients. I don't mean the ones they choose for you; I mean for them to allow you to choose whichever patient you would like to speak to. The bottom line is this: gamma knife is very expensive, and many insurance companies will not pay for it. It runs in the range of fifty thousand dollars, depending on where you have it done.

I know of two people who had it done for brain tumors, and it did not work for either of them. For one person it made the tumor grow faster, and the other was paralyzed by it. Both had to do it more than one time. Instead of blasting your entire head with a low dose of radiation over a seven-week period, they focus on your tumor with the setting on full blast. This extreme-dose focus on a small area is very dangerous if the intended target is missed. I recommend staying clear of this option, but of course, investigate it yourself and make your own judgment.

7

Health Insurance Must Change

I don't understand the logic used by health insurance companies. I asked the cancer center how much of my one-million-dollar health insurance benefit was going to be used up by the seven-week radiation program. Of course, they fiddled around, pretending as if they didn't know exactly how much it cost. They do radiation all year round and they don't know what it costs? NOT!

I've seen many cases where these places bleed your insurance dry. When it is all gone, then they say, "Sorry, we tried all we could. Go home and enjoy your remaining time with your family, there's nothing else we can do."

The response they gave me regarding the cost was, "Don't worry, your insurance will cover it, and if it doesn't, Medicare will cover it. I can find out for you later." This is what they told me, and later never came. The only thing that came later was a bill for two fifteen-minute simulations to the toll of over two thousand dollars.

That was only the simulations. I could only imagine what seven weeks of radiation would come out to.

I just don't understand it. If I was an insurance company, I would rather spend five to ten thousand dollars on an alternative cancer treatment that would bring the patient back to health fast, so I wouldn't have to pay out large amounts for a long period. As opposed to paying two to three hundred thousand on conventional therapies that make the patients sicker and don't work.

Why should we be forced to take a treatment that we do not agree with because it is the only treatment the insurance company will pay for? Don't we have the right to choose the type of treatment we feel most comfortable with? Many people cannot afford to go the natural route. They have no choice but to do the treatment that the doctors and insurance companies will pay for. This is unfair, especially since you are the one paying the premiums. If they would cover patients who chose the alternative therapies, it would force many of the doctors that do conventional treatments to look for a better way to cure cancer.

The keyword here is *cure*, not to increase survival by so many years. Other keywords are *prevention* and *education*. We need to educate our people so serious illnesses can be prevented. With the brightest minds and the most resources of any country in the world, we could find the cure for cancer if we really wanted to. This country put its mind to go to the moon, something people only dreamed about for centuries. We did it in less than ten years. God has blessed this great nation of ours with everything we need to be a world leader.

So when are we going to put the profits aside and let our conscience do what is right? Let's eliminate all the obstacles that are in the way of this achievable goal. The way things are now, if there is research money for how to stop pimples from growing, the universities will research pimples. Instead, they should be researching alternatives for cancer that show promise.

We must have some sort of political change in our healthcare system. It should be a gradual change, not a radical change, because people are afraid of that. Since I am on the subject of change, I would like to address the politicians out there. First, I would like to say that anyone can get cancer. It could be yourself, your wife, kids, mother, father, uncle, etc. I want to tell you a personal story, because people do not see or notice problems until they happen to them.

The year was 1985. I was in my one-room efficiency with my wife, Elizabeth. At the time, we didn't have health insurance. We were trying hard to have a baby, and Elizabeth had a miscarriage at thirteen weeks three months prior. Now she was pregnant again, and again at thirteen weeks she began to spot. She went to the gynecologist and he ordered her on bedrest. For a month, Elizabeth only got up to go to the bathroom. She was trying desperately to hold on to this child. When I saw that it was a losing battle, I had to carry her to the car and go to the nearest hospital. Elizabeth was bleeding profusely, and I feared for her life. I had to carry her into the emergency room with blood everywhere.

"My wife needs help, she is losing the baby," I told the receptionist.

"Do you have insurance?" she asked.

"No! I do not," I said.

"Well, she's going to have to go to the county hospital to do a D&C."

I was in shock! How could anyone say that when there is a life-threatening condition like that? I was extremely upset and argued with them until they agreed to stabilize her, but they needed to call an ambulance and transfer her right away. When the ambulance arrived, I was in for another shock.

"You don't have insurance, so you're going to have to pay cash before we take her."

What in the world was going on here? I was in my shorts and sandals having rushed out of the house to save my wife's life—I didn't take cash with me. How could we treat our own people with such little sensitivity and value? If Elizabeth was the wife of some congressman or senator, they would not have treated her like this. Why do we put more value on people who are fortunate than those who are unfortunate? Aren't we all equal in God's eyes? No one knows how this treatment feels unless you experience it yourself. My dad had to come and bring me $145 for a ten-minute drive to the county hospital. A cab would have been only $8.

We need a real leader who will commit as Kennedy did. This time, let it be to find a *cure* for cancer in ten years. People who are suffering can't wait. Their lives depend on it.

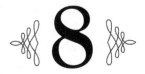

Fight for Your Work Benefits

Hopefully, you'll have a job that provides benefits. Not everyone does. If you're one of the lucky ones like I was, you'll still need to fight to make sure you receive what's yours. Insurance companies do not like to pay, and employers will do their best to get rid of you. When they find out that you're sick, they don't want anything to do with you and will try to eliminate you from their payroll as soon as possible.

You need to once again skip all the middlemen and go to the director of human resources. Shortly after I returned home, I went to my work and made the mistake of not going to the top. I brought along a nurse friend of mine to help me understand all the benefits that I was entitled to. They like to make everything very complicated so you won't understand it. In this way, you might slip through a crack and not fill out a particular form or miss a deadline for continuing coverage.

This person was very insensitive to my predicament and was also very rude. I asked her to please explain to me all my benefits.

"I already explained them to your wife and brother and answered their questions." This was her way of greeting me.

"Well, obviously you didn't answer all of their questions, or else I wouldn't be here," I told her.

This person was notorious for not being helpful in any way, shape, or form, and maybe that's why she was in that position. She was excellent at keeping the employees in the dark about their benefits.

She began to explain my benefits in her usual manner that no one understood and not allowing you to interrupt to ask any questions.

"Can you please explain what you just said?" I asked.

"Are you going to be interrupting me with questions, or are you going to let me continue?" she barked at me.

"I hope you don't mind, but I need to record this conversation because I'm having problems remembering things since my surgery." She didn't object, but you could see in her eyes that this made her very uncomfortable.

As she proceeded, I interrupted one more time because she was very confusing. That's when she really ticked me off.

"Does he understand what's going on?" she whispered to my nurse friend who was with me.

I looked at her and said, "Yes, I understand perfectly, it's you that is not explaining yourself correctly, and if you had three kids and no income, you would want to know everything too!"

"Calm down, Jimmy, I'll take care of this," my friend said to me.

I'm not supposed to get upset, and it seems everywhere I've turned, trying to claim my rights, a brick wall was slapped in my face. Thank God that Miriam came with me. She's the one that drove me there. I couldn't drive anymore because of the possibility of a seizure. Once I went over this person's head, I didn't have any more trouble. As a matter of fact, they were very helpful and understanding.

9

The Spiritual: Many Rivers to the Same Ocean

Spirituality is very important. I believe when you have cancer, you already have two strikes against you. Not believing in God as your creator might as well be strike three. People too many times search for answers in man and the material world.

Many times, nonbelievers don't do as well as a person who believes in God and prays. Those with faith seem more at peace with themselves. They also seem to recover faster and more often. I believe God will help all who seek His help. He answers all prayers that come from the heart. At least from my experience, He has answered all of my prayers. I don't feel worthy of this honor. I had faith that God would heal me, and He did. Every time I go to church and I eat the body and blood of Christ, I thank the Lord for another day of living.

Then I say a little prayer that goes like this:

Thank you, Lord, for allowing me to live one more week and to be honored to participate in the eating of Your healing body and blood. Thank you, Lord, for Your healing blood. I pray that Your healing blood, which is more powerful than any doctor's medicine, travels directly to my tumor and eliminates any remaining tumor cells that may be there. I also pray that You heal all the sick in the way You have healed me. Thank you, Lord, and guide me in the right direction.

41

After saying this prayer, I feel confident that I will be back next week.

Religion is slightly different from the spiritual. I don't like to get into religion too much because I am very weak in this subject. I was raised a Catholic and have recently been baptized in the Church of Christ as a Christian. I would like to say that I have discovered all the answers, but I'd be lying. I feel that due to cultural differences in the world there will always be different ways that people worship God. Because of these cultural differences, it would be virtually impossible for everyone to believe the same thing in their pursuit to serve God.

I don't believe that one religion is right, and another is wrong. As long as a person believes in one God and lives a life of love for their fellow man, I think they will reach heaven. If you look at the earth from space, you will see many rivers that lead to the same ocean. I see them representing different religions and cultures; they all take different paths and turns, but in the end, they all end up draining into the same ocean, which I see as heaven.

All of God's children that seek the truth will find it. I believe the more spiritually evolved you are, the more tolerant one becomes of different religions. Whoever is good at heart is on the right track to God. I don't understand how all the religions of the world speak about God and are always fighting with their neighbors about who is right and who's wrong. This has been a curse on mankind.

If we all accepted our differences and practiced what we preach of our own religions, we would all live in harmony and peace. Why must we fight over stupid things as if we were children? I sometimes listen to my three children argue and fight over the dumbest things that are not important. I'm sure God is in heaven looking down at the world and saying the same thing about us. As a parent, I know exactly what God is thinking: stop fighting and arguing over silly things and concentrate on loving one another, because you are all brothers and sisters and are all my children.

It pains me to see my children when they fight, and I'm sure it pains God as well. **God is in every one of us, so when you hurt someone you're hurting God.** There is only one God, and He is worshipped in many different ways depending on the culture they were raised in. I believe that Jesus Christ is my Lord and Savior and He died on the cross to remove the sins of the world, and that includes all of mankind. I have been blessed to know of Him and to have experienced His presence, but I don't see how an Indian in the middle of the Amazon Rainforest would be condemned to hell because he has never heard of Jesus Christ or been baptized. Fighting amongst each other over religion throughout the centuries has brought nothing but hardship to this world. Not until we put our differences aside and face the reality that we are *all* equally God's children and a part of him will peace come to this beleaguered world of ours. It is very important that we love God by treating one another in the same way we would treat Him.

It's so simple. Look at your enemy and see the God you love standing in front of you. Are you going to strike him down, or are you going to embrace him? It's your decision. We will all find ourselves in this position one day with someone we do not like. God will constantly test us to see how we respond.

I may be wrong about this, but as I said, I am not an expert on religion. There are many things that I do not understand. It doesn't seem fair, and *I* believe God is an all-loving God who is fair and would not allow that to happen.

We are all spiritually connected, and the sooner we all understand that, the sooner we'll have peace on earth.

When I left the hospital, I was very depressed and confused. I didn't know which way to turn for help. I only knew one thing: if my choices were to put my life in the hands of the doctors or the hands of God, I would without question go with God. I am not an expert on God or religion. I only know and say what I feel in my heart.

If you want to find your happiness, just look for someone who is really hurting and in need and help them.

One time my wife was driving me home when I saw an accident; it was a minor fender bender. The only thing out of the ordinary was this very young girl who was kneeling on the ground in the pouring rain crying her eyes out in the middle of the street.

My first thought was, *What is this girl doing there? She's going to get killed if she doesn't get out of there.* Since I couldn't drive, and my wife was in a hurry to get back to work, I didn't say anything. On the way home all I could think of was that Jesus was back there crying in the middle of the street.

Once I got home, without hesitation, I picked up my checkbook and told my two boys to put their raincoats on because we were going for a walk. We walked almost a half-mile back in the pouring rain because I felt this was not only another chance to help God but also a tremendous opportunity to teach my boys a lesson on helping others. I took my time, because I knew that when I arrived there, everything would be exactly the same.

God knew I was coming with good intentions and there was a lesson to be taught. Of course, the young girl was still kneeling on the ground staring at her bumper. I asked her, "Is there anything I could do for you?"

"No! I'm finished, I don't know what I'm going to do."

I looked at the bumper and couldn't understand why she was so upset; there was barely a dent on the bumper. What appeared to me as nothing was like the end of the world to her. For whatever reason, this was a traumatic event for her. So traumatic that she had risked her life kneeling in front of her car in the rain with slippery roads and just after a curve in the road. I knew that I had to convince her to get off the street and out of harm's way.

"It's not that bad. You should try getting the car out of the way and get out of the rain."

"It is bad, this is a 1967. I'll never find a bumper to replace it," she cried.

The police arrived and made her move the car to a side street. I understood because of her tender age of sixteen all of this was very terrifying to her. The only way I felt that I could relieve her grief was to help her financially. She appeared to be a very responsible sixteen-year-old. She was dressed in a fast-food uniform. I knew by looking at the broken-down 1967 car, and the fact that she was working at sixteen, that she was not that well off. This may have had a lot to do with her grief.

I told her to calm down. "The car is only a material object and is not that important." She started to cry. She told me that her uncle bought her the car for three hundred dollars, and if she damaged it he would not fix it and the car would rot in front of the house. It was her only transportation to work, where she worked only twelve hours on the weekend. At this point, I wrote a check for two hundred dollars and gave it to her.

"Here, take this check. I know it's not much, but it should help you fix the car."

She began to cry hysterically. "What are you doing? You don't even know me," she kept repeating over and over. "How could you do this?" It was beyond her comprehension that someone would come out of nowhere to help her.

Unfortunately, that's the way our society is today. I would be in shock too. We need to get away from this "fend for yourself" mentality. I told her that I've been helped by many people I didn't know and this was my way of paying them back.

"It doesn't matter whether you know someone. When someone is in need, you should help them," I told her. I was going to tell her that I did know her, that she was my sister, but she would not have understood. I told her that God works in mysterious ways. I knew this would be an experience she would never forget. I'm sure she would tell many people about her experience. Someday, when she is older and finds herself in a position to help someone, she won't even hesitate. The more people she tells, the better chance that a domino effect of kindness to others will occur.

The seeds we plant today are the flowers of tomorrow. I told my wife, so she could balance the checkbook. She must have thought I was crazy, especially knowing the financial situation we were in. I was not working and the hospital bills were piling up daily. She understood perfectly and just told me jokingly that she was going to hide the checkbook.

My two boys learned a lesson on helping others. I teach them to help the poor by giving them some money so they can give it to the homeless person and experience the joy of giving. We all love our family and friends. It's not until we are at the brink that we realize our relationship with God is the most important thing in life.

In the end, it's only you and God. I recommend that everyone have children. By having children or being with children, one can understand easier the relationship we all have with our Father in Heaven. God loves us all in the same way we love our children.

Ever since I was a child, I felt I had a personal relationship with Jesus Christ.

When I was a child, I would ask my father to go and play outside with my friends. I would leave the warmth and safety of my comfortable home to go out to play. I would be so involved in having fun with my friends that I would sometimes forget I even had a father and a warm home.

This is what happens to us all in life. We leave our home in heaven to come and play on earth. We are so distracted by what we're doing on earth that we forget that we have a wonderful father and beautiful home to come back to. When my father would call me to come home, I never wanted to go home. I was playing with my friends that I loved and didn't want to leave them. That's the same thing that happens with life on earth. We are reluctant to leave the people we know and love.

Finally, when I would come home, I realized that it was my father who loved me the most. This is the same in real life. When you have a near-death experience is when you realize that it's your fellowship with God that is the most important thing in life. A good friend from my Little League team asked me if I would go with her to her church because they have all been praying for me. She was afraid to ask, not knowing what religion I practiced.

I said of course I'd go; I will thank anyone that has been praying for me no matter what religion. I went to this church that I was totally unfamiliar with. I didn't ask what denomination they were; I figured as long as they pray to God, I'm okay. It was the type of mass where people get up to dance and sing praises to the Lord. I felt strange and out of place, but I joined in as much as I could.

I was very weak and began to get very emotional even though I could barely understand what they were saying. The mass was in Spanish, and even though I do speak Spanish, I was born in New Jersey and my Spanish vocabulary is limited to that of an elementary-school level. Every time I would look at the cross on the altar, tears would run down my face. I don't know why; I just couldn't do anything about it.

There was a part where people who were sick could come up and ask to be healed, so I went up. I was caught up in the emotion of the moment. I asked Jesus to heal me, and they asked me if I believed Jesus was my savior. "Yes," I replied with all my heart. I knew that I would heal before I went there, and this reassured me that Jesus would heal me or guide me in the right direction so that I could be healed.

Another person whom I believe had a lot to do with my recovery is one of the greatest people alive: my father, Antonio Blanco. I believe he has a direct connection with God. He has an insight on everything in life that, by far, surpasses anyone that I have ever met in my life. I'm not saying this because he's my dad. I love him and think highly of him, as most people do about their own dads. There truly is something special and holy about him. He is so confident and knowledgeable about everything in life that you feel like you're in good hands.

I believe that it was his special influence with God that saved me in surgery.

I began to attend the church at the private Christian school where my children go to school. There, I experienced the same feelings I had encountered in the other church. I could not stop the tears from flowing whenever I would look at the cross. I would also get very emotional when songs of praise were sung. It's so hard to explain. It's like when you were a kid trying to learn how to read. You can't get it; you keep trying and trying, and then suddenly it just kicks in and you finally understand it.

All the meanings of the songs just kicked in. The message behind each song was coming in loud and clear, and this caused me to weep with joy and sorrow. This service was also strange to me because I was raised a Catholic. I don't limit myself in my search for truth and knowledge. I was baptized in the Church of Christ and I continue to attend service on Sunday.

TRUST. IN. GOD.

When tragedy falls upon us and our loved ones, it is difficult to understand. We become upset and ask God, why have you done this to me? I am beginning to understand now with the help of children.

I recently managed my son Jason's Little League baseball team. We were playing a very good team. Nelson, the real manager, went on vacation and entrusted me to win this very important game. I studied the opposing team for two weeks to plan my strategy on how to beat them. I knew exactly where to position my players for each one of their players. During the game, my son became very upset with me.

He was playing pitcher and standing on the right side of the pitcher's mound. When I saw who was batting, I switched him to the left side of the mound. The ball was hit hard through the right side, precisely where he was standing. He was mad and asked me, "Dad, why did you move me? I would have had it!"

I knew what I was doing, and I had anticipated that happening. I remember my state of mind at the time. I told him he didn't need to know why I did it, he just had to trust me and do what I told him. I am the manager and I do what I do to win the game.

"I don't need to explain anything. You just need to know that it was for the good of the team." He stayed upset for the rest of the game. I knew that the batter was going to hit the ball on the right side of the pitcher's mound, because I had tracked this player's hitting for the past seven games and ninety percent of the time he would hit it to the shortstop.

Even though I knew my son was a very good player, I also knew that the ball would be hit very hard and he would not have enough time to react and would most probably deflect it and the batter would get on base. By moving him to the left side, the ball would be hit right to my shortstop, who has a cannon for an arm and would easily get him out. That's exactly what happened, just as I'd planned.

At the end of the game, my son Jason was still frustrated because he couldn't understand why I did what I did. I began to reflect. Isn't this how we all feel when tragedy occurs to us that we can't understand? We are always asking God, why did you do that, or why did this have to happen? God is the big manager in heaven and we are all players on His team.

When what we perceive as a tragedy happens to us, we should not ask why. We don't need to know why. We must trust in God that whatever happened was for the good of the team in his plan to win the game. The team is all of us. When loved ones pass away, consider it similar to a sacrifice bunt. In baseball, we sometimes ask a player to bunt the ball, knowing that he is going to be out, but also knowing that he bunted the potential winning run over to second base. We didn't want him to be out, but sacrificed the batter anyway to win the game. The point is to trust in God. That's what our founding fathers placed on our currency—"In God We Trust"—right? He is looking out for us all; we are on His team and God plays to win.

When I was discharged from the hospital, I was depressed and confident at the same time. Depressed because the doctors had just told me that I had a terminal illness that has no cure, and confident that God would guide me in the right direction so that I may be cured. I was only given two options by the medical establishment: one, chemotherapy; and two, radiation. Neither one would cure me, only prolong my life for a short period. I went to the cancer center like every other patient. I prepared to begin radiation. They made a special mask for me and told me I was to begin the following Monday.

I knew that I only had a few days to decide whether to go ahead with the radiation. A friend of mine from work, Isabell, was really the one who started the ball rolling in the right direction. She gave me the telephone number of a cancer survivor and I went to see her. I was new at this, but she knew what I was going through.

She talked to me about the terrible mistake she had made by taking radiation therapy. She described how the radiation burned her esophagus and how it took her a year just to recover from the radiation. She vowed never to put herself through that again. She talked about how she improved by changing her diet and how she had been in remission for ten years.

For the first time, I began to see some hope. It seemed strange that it was just a regular person and not a physician that was giving me this hope. I took a walk in the mall, walking with my wife, praying for a sign on what I should do. We entered a bookstore and my wife showed me a book by Dr. William Lane called *Sharks Don't Get Cancer*. I found the topic interesting, so I bought it and began to read it. When the day came for me to begin radiation, I called the cancer center and asked for another week to think about it.

I naturally have a very inquisitive personality. I never take anyone's word and always find things out for myself. I also have the personality of always taking the opposite point of view to the majority opinion on almost all topics. I do this just to prove people wrong or get their reactions. I began to educate myself as much as I could about brain cancer. At the same time, I prayed a lot and went to church. Whatever church that I was invited to, I would go. I concentrated on having a positive mind.

I strongly believe that your mind is so powerful that if you think negatively, you will experience negative results and get sicker. If you think positively, you will experience positive results and get well.

I was invited to go to a hypnotist by Diane. She helped me to meditate and think positively, and she also helped me with visualization. Visualization is a very powerful tool in eliminating illness. I would use visualization before I even knew what it was. I would visualize myself small enough to be inside my brain and I would be shooting the tumor with a ray gun.

Whenever I would do an MRI, the noise made by the machine sounded to me like the drills workers use to break cement. I would visualize myself using one of these drills to break my tumor apart.

I also was convinced that I had to change my diet forever. I am not a doctor and I recommend everyone is monitored by a physician while doing conventional or alternative therapies. I do not think there are any magic bullets out there that will cure cancer. The alternative that is good for you will depend on the type of cancer you have. I think it is a combination of modalities that does the trick.

Choosing a good nutritionist will be very important, even though I didn't have one. They were too expensive for me and I never found one that was willing to give free advice. You must be willing to change your eating habits forever. Good nutrition is very important to reestablish your health. Everyone is different; what works for one person may not work for another. You must be flexible and be ready to change treatment or add supplements to your treatment. I can only tell you what I did.

When you venture out into the unknown, and I say unknown because the average person has never even heard about alternative treatments, you may not find the answers to your questions right away. Be patient, you will see how one thing leads to another. The more networking you do, the better. The more people you talk to, the more you will learn, and before you know it, you will not remember where you started unless you kept notes. Documentation and records of everything you have done are very important. This is very difficult to do when the information begins to come in faster than you can keep track of. Make a special effort to keep good records. They will benefit you as you progress.

❧ 10 ❧

My Journey Begins

My journey began when I picked up the book *Sharks Don't Get Cancer* by Dr. William Lane. I found it amazing. The concept was so simple that it bewildered me that it was not being used by the medical establishment. As I understand it, tumor cells need new blood vessels to grow. The proteins found in the cartilage of the shark apparently inhibit the growth of new blood vessels needed by the tumor to grow. There are many different ailments that shark cartilage is good for other than the prevention of tumor growth, treatments for osteoarthritis being one of them.

I will bet anything that the pharmaceutical companies are in their laboratories right now trying to figure out a way to synthesize shark cartilage to sell it as a drug. Why make a drug out of something that is natural and already available?

God gave man everything he needs, and it is all in nature. I believe the cure for every disease can be found in nature. I just hope that we find the answers before all the rainforests are destroyed. Economically speaking, I do not think it is in the best interest of the doctors and hospitals to educate the public on simple and economical treatments for cancers. They would lose money for sure; I know they lost money on me. I had a one-million-dollar limit on my health insurance. They could have easily persuaded me to spend two to three hundred thousand dollars on chemotherapy and radiation if I didn't know any better.

Believe me, they tried. The scare tactics are their best chance of hooking you, and they usually work. You have three months to live, so don't take too long in deciding, even though it will not save you anyhow.

Without these new blood vessels the tumor needs so desperately, it can no longer grow and eventually becomes necrotic and dies. I could not believe that Dr. Lane had to go outside this country to do his research. He used his own money to fund his research. For someone to be using his own money, he was coming from the heart. There is so much greed in the medical profession that it is pitiful. Why do doctors have this need to be so rich? What they should be doing is more charity work for the patients that do not have insurance and cannot pay for their services.

When you find a physician that cares more about restoring you to health rather than who your insurance provider is, then you have found a real doctor you can trust.

I rushed to the health food store to buy some shark cartilage.

Buyer beware! You will come across people in health food stores who are honest and sincere, then some are profiteers and dishonest. These people pass themselves off as experts in areas they know nothing about. I learned that the hard way.

I was in a desperate race with time, since I was only given three months to live. In my desperation, I listened to the proprietor, who appeared knowledgeable in this field, and I purchased seven injectable vials of shark cartilage. They each cost twenty-seven dollars, and I was told to take two a day. They told me that my case demanded extreme measures.

I went home very happy with my vials, but I thought to myself, *What do I do with them now that I have them?* I managed to track down where Dr. Lane's office in New Jersey was and called. I asked the secretary about shark cartilage.

"I purchased six vials of shark cartilage and don't know how to inject them."

"Inject?" she replied. "Can you hold on, please?"

After a long wait, a man came on the phone extremely upset.

"What do you mean, inject? Take those vials and throw them

in the garbage! They're nothing but sugar water and are absolutely worthless! I can't believe these people are making a mockery of my work!"

I could not believe that I actually had the famous Dr. Lane on the other end of the phone.

God was truly guiding me in the right direction. He spoke to me and cleared up many of my questions. Any shark cartilage other than BeneFin is not the cartilage that has been tested in clinical trials throughout the world. BeneFin is specially made in Australia. The product is never touched by the human hand. This process makes it a safer product compared to how they are processed by other companies out there.

Despite having a good idea of how to use the product, I continued to search for a doctor that has used shark cartilage on real patients. I came up with a man named Dr. Dante Ruccio in New Jersey. When I called him, I wasn't expecting much, but I received a lot. I spoke to him personally for one hour and he made a lot of sense. He appeared to be speaking from the heart and seemed to be a very caring man. He made a point that really hit home: he asked me how much money I spent on my last office visit.

I said, "Two hundred and fifty dollars."

Then he asked, "How much time did the doctor spend with you?"

"Ten to fifteen minutes tops," I answered.

"Well, I just spent one hour with you without charging you a dime. I just want you to get well."

This told me a lot about the man. This is how all doctors should be. They should be concerned more for their patients. A large majority of doctors only worry about how much money they make from the insurance company before they die. They also try to figure out ways they can keep you returning for office visits. A doctor's worst nightmare is that the public becomes aware of all the helpful alternatives out there. Especially since they know nothing about them.

I see a nationwide trend where more and more people are

asking for alternatives as opposed to conventional therapies. People are asking their doctors about these alternatives, and all they can comment on is that it's hogwash. They are not educated on alternatives and do not want to be educated.

Keep looking until you find the right healthcare provider for you.

The only time a doctor will venture out into the alternative arena is when one of their family members is afflicted with an incurable disease. Dr. Lane mentioned that when he visited Positive Alternative Therapies in Health, Inc., in Miami. He also stated that a very high percentage of doctors take antioxidants but would never prescribe them to their patients.

I sent out for the BeneFin shark cartilage along with other products Dr. Ruccio suggested I take, but there was a problem. It had only been a couple of weeks since my surgery. It is not recommended to take shark cartilage so soon after surgery. It's recommended to wait four to six weeks, but I was in a race with time. I had to weigh the pros and cons concerning my situation. If I waited that long, I was taking the chance of the tumor regrowing to a very large size. If I took the shark cartilage too soon, I was taking the chance that the brain would not heal properly.

Dr. Ruccio and I discussed it and he suggested I start with a small amount of six grams every other day for a few weeks. I started on November 22, 1995, just twenty-two days after surgery.

I accidentally took twenty-four grams in one dose because my wife and I didn't know what we were doing. Then I took three grams twice a day, every other day. A week later I increased the dosage to six grams twice a day, every other day.

Dr. Lane suggests 1.2 grams per kilo of body weight. One kilo equals 2.2 pounds, so for me, I calculated 81 grams was all right for me. Dr. Ruccio suggested 96 grams.

The day before my follow-up visit with my neurosurgeon, I did an MRI to see if the tumor was growing. I went to the doctor's office and he asked me what I was doing for my condition as far as chemotherapy and radiation.

I told him nothing, because I decided against any such treatments. He told me not to totally rule out radiation and reconsider because my condition is very serious. I said to him, "Why don't you call the hospital and have them fax the MRI results over and we will check them out together and decide on a course of action."

He received the fax and read it to himself in front of me, and it seemed forever.

"Well, what does it say?"

"It says there is no tumor growth," he responded in a somewhat surprised manner. Those words were music to my ears.

I said to myself, "Thank you, Lord."

The doctor asked me, "So when are you going back to work?"

I wish I could, but I was suffering from many symptoms that still seriously limit my activities. Some of these symptoms included seizures, back pain, short-term memory loss, loss of train of thought, mental and physical fatigue requiring frequent naps, poor sleep due to constant urination and needing to have my head elevated, poor grip, the feeling of electricity and twitching in my extremities, a constant itch that must have been inside my skull near the incision site, and constant headaches of which there were four kinds: stabbing, burning, pressure, and bone pain headaches. The pressure headaches are the worst. The only way I could describe it is for you to place your thumb on your temple and press in as hard as you can until you can't stand the pain, then leave the pressure on all day long.

I began with the products Dr. Ruccio suggested for my particular cancer, plus I continued to research on my own. I added any herb that was good for the brain and the repair of brain tissue. As long as they didn't have any side effects like drugs do, I was game. I also began to wean myself off a steroid and drug for acid indigestion. You should never abruptly stop taking any medications. One should always wean slowly and with a physician monitoring you at all times.

The only medication I didn't mess with was my anti-seizure medication, because this would prevent seizures. The doctors say

I must remain on this drug for the rest of my life. Excuse me if I don't think so. It will be a great challenge for me to wean myself off this drug that is harmful to the liver.

I started taking the herbs echinacea, Vital Veggies, Earth Source Greens & More, Cat's Claw, ImmunoFin, Ester-c with bioflavonoids, Phytaid, shark cartilage, flaxseed oil, astragalus, CoQ10, Advanced Antioxidant Formula, a daily multivitamin, an anabolic recovery and nutrition powder for athletes, and Myrrh-Goldenseal Plus.

I spoke to Dr. Ruccio in early December a few weeks later and told him my MRI results, and he asked me to go immediately to ninety-six grams of shark cartilage.

Due to my inability to do many things for myself, I found it very difficult to mix four drinks a day of twenty-four grams. My wife, Elizabeth, was the one doing everything for me. She also had the three children and work to attend to. She managed to make three drinks of fresh organic carrots combined with either apple, oranges, lettuce, cabbage, beets, or cucumbers.

Elizabeth made many different combinations using the book *Raw Vegetable Juices* by N. W. Walker, DSc. This change in diet is essential for anyone's recovery. I was always a meat and potato guy. Since I never had time to cook, many times all I ate was fast food. Now, I call those fast-food places "murderer's row" because they are always lined up one after the other and serve what I consider poison to the public.

I had never even tasted a carrot before. I was disgusted by the taste and I still am. By changing my diet, I lost thirty-five pounds. I am five foot four and weighed 175 pounds when I got sick. That was too much, so I dropped to a normal body weight of 140 pounds. I had been overweight for twelve years and tried many starvation diets to take it off. It never worked, and I experienced what some people call the yo-yo effect. I always gained all my weight back and then some. I believe these herbs increased my metabolism, because I lost weight without even trying.

The more research I did, the more herbs I would add. I bought the book *Prescription for Nutritional Healing* by James and Phyllis Balch. This is a very helpful book for someone interested in using natural remedies. It is a reference guide to many different conditions from A to Z using vitamins, minerals, herbs, and food supplements.

Many people with good intentions would give me certain products. If they had no side effects and made sense to me, I would add them. I knew my liver was the most important organ to keep healthy. I added grape root drops that are supposed to be good for the liver. I added herbal teas and also added Triple Garlic, garlic being a natural antibiotic. Later I discovered that aged garlic was a better product and switched to it.

I added Myrrh-Goldenseal Plus, which is an herb good for many ailments. Melatonin I began using because of all the publicity that had come out during the time. I began to use it but stopped because it would stay in my system for days. It made me feel very weak and tired, more than I already was. I only use it when I absolutely could not sleep or if I was going to have an MRI. One was more than enough.

At this time, I was also weaning myself slowly off my prescribed medications of ranitidine for acid indigestion and the corticosteroid dexamethasone. According to Dr. Ruccio, dexamethasone is good, but it can also be bad when used for prolonged periods. It is good to reduce swelling after surgery, but two months later I was still on very high doses, for what reason I don't know. Dexamethasone can also cause edema in my brain, which can cause pressure. This is just as bad as a tumor; the pressure could push on the brain and create seizures.

Looking back, in retrospect, many of these supplements might not have been necessary. I did them all because I felt like a pioneer in unfamiliar waters. I hope that my experience can be refined so that others may do just as well without taking unnecessary pills. The reason I mention everything I did is because it worked that way for me. You must remember I am not a doctor, so use your own judgment and ask for professional advice.

I continued to add products: ginseng and bee pollen, lecithin,

Kyo-Green Drink, ginkgo biloba, chickweed, blessed thistle, fenugreek, an enzyme support supplement, parsley leaf, and aloe vera.

I was now in a war against a fierce enemy, and if you ask any general, they will tell you the way to win a war is with overwhelming force. The more firepower one has, the better chance they have of winning the war. This is the mental state that I was in. I refused to be beaten by this puny invader of my body.

After a month of taking all these pills, I became concerned about my liver. Could my liver handle it all? I knew a healthy liver was vital for my recovery. Prescription drugs such as my anti-seizure medication may cause liver damage. Also, the number of pills I was taking motivated me to do more research on how best to avoid any liver problems. The liver makes bile that helps with digestion. It detoxifies all the bad things we ingest. It stores energy. It manufactures proteins. It stores vitamins and minerals. Your liver should be soft and smooth, not hard and bumpy.

In the book *Prescription for Nutritional Healing*, the herb milk thistle is a very potent liver protector, and it stimulates new liver cell production. I was very cautious and began taking just one a day.

I kept very good records of everything that I was taking with exact times. I separated the pills that were to be taken with meals and those with an empty stomach. If it weren't for my lovely wife, Elizabeth, who did everything for me, I don't know where I'd be. I was too weak, dizzy, and with terrible headaches to do anything for myself.

I took a blend of digestive and systemic enzymes along with daily fiber to keep me regular. Regular bowel movement is very important, and I felt worse when I was not regular.

I had a lot of trouble sleeping. I needed my head elevated, my headaches were unbearable, and I'd be drenched in sweat. It was so bad that I had to sleep with two or three towels underneath me. I needed to wake up every hour or two to urinate. I would lose my grip on objects. My short-term memory was really bad; I would begin a conversation and forget where I started. I was in pretty bad shape. I think the single most important ingredient was the will to live. That's what it comes down to. My three beautiful children—Jamie, nine; Jimmy Jr., eight; and Jason, six—were my motivation to go on and not quit.

Two and a half months into my treatment, I picked up the book *The Cure for All Cancers* by Hulda Regehr Clark. Her theory, as I understood it, was that all cancers are caused by a single parasite called the human intestinal fluke. If the parasite is killed, the cancer will be gone. When the parasite remains in the intestines, you may be saved, but once they migrate to the liver, according to Clark, it causes cancer. According to her book, one hundred percent of all cancer patients have two things in common: they have propyl alcohol and the intestinal fluke in their liver.

Now, remember, I was desperately looking for answers and had nothing to lose in trying anything. I decided to add her program to my regimen. My battle plan was set. First, I was to cut off the enemy supply line by not using any products that contained the letters "prop" together. This included propyl alcohol, propanol, isopropanol, and propylene glycol. I checked the labels on everything from foods to cosmetics.

Second, I would begin to use the three herbs she suggested in her book. The black walnut hull tincture are drops and are supposed to kill the adult fluke. The wormwood capsule, these are pills and are supposed to kill the four in-between stages of the fluke. The cloves is probably the most important; it is supposed to kill the eggs. I began using these herbs, in addition to my barrage of other herbs, minerals, vitamins, amino acids, enzymes, and most important, shark cartilage. I also took L-Ornithine and Arginine. These amino acids would help counter the release of ammonia that is the parasite's waste product.

Hulda Regehr Clark's book states that the flukes will be dead by day five. I began on January 16, 1996, and on the twelfth day I became very sick and was taken to the hospital. I had a dramatic and deeply spiritual event happen in that emergency room, but I'll expand on that a little later. After coming home, I discovered what appeared to be hundreds of parasites in my stool that looked identical to the flukes shown in the book.

I theorized that perhaps the release of ammonia from thousands of dead parasites at the same time may have been the cause of my symptoms that landed me in the hospital. In retrospect, maybe if I had also been taking an herbal laxative after day four, this large accumulation of ammonia would not have occurred. I am only guessing and speculating, because this is only my theory. Then again, these herbs may have been the cause of my problem that day. I don't know. I stay away from the propyl alcohol products to be on the safe side, but I also stopped taking these herbs.

NOTE: Author of *The Cure for All Cancers*, Hulda Clark, faced a series of lawsuits by the US Federal Trade Commission after her central claims were thoroughly debunked. She relocated to Mexico, where she set up a cancer clinic, but she died of multiple myeloma, a blood cancer, in 2009.

11

Shark Cartilage

The shark cartilage product is what I believe was the single most important supplement I took. I've exclusively taken the BeneFin product. Before taking this product, you should consult with an experienced professional. Caution must be taken if you are pregnant, nursing, recovering from surgery, or have a heart or circulatory condition. I started slowly because I just had major brain surgery. The body needs to recover; it is best to wait a while before taking the shark cartilage. A few weeks should do the trick. The theory is that the shark cartilage inhibits the growth of new blood vessels (anti-angiogenesis) needed by the tumors to grow. By eliminating these new blood vessels, you can eventually cut off the tumor's blood supply. This will cause the tumor to become necrotic and die.

I began about three weeks after surgery with small doses. After another week I increased the dose to twenty-five grams three times a day for a total of seventy-five grams. In Dr. Lane's book, *Sharks Don't Get Cancer*, he suggests 1.2 grams of dry cartilage per one kilogram (2.2 pounds) of body weight to inhibit rapidly growing tumors. I weighed 150 pounds, or 68.18 kilograms (1.2 x 68.18 = 81.81 g). I knew Dr. Ruccio suggested I take ninety-six grams, but my wife, who was doing them for me, didn't have time to do it four times a day, so I managed only three. Dr. Ruccio will be very angry with me if he reads this book, because he really cares and doesn't want me to fail.

Shark cartilage decreases the ability of abnormal blood vessels to grow, leaving the normal blood vessels alone. I say abnormal because they are growing in a location where they should not be. As I understand it, tumors are accompanied by abnormal blood vessels.

These abnormal blood vessels are what the shark cartilage targets. The only time our bodies create new blood vessels is when we have surgery, when a woman is pregnant, or when a tumor is growing. That is why it is not recommended to be taken while pregnant or after surgery.

I took seventy-five grams religiously for two months and then dropped to fifty grams. I did this on my own; Dr. Ruccio will suggest a longer time and I would recommend you listen to him. I was using myself as a living guinea pig to see if I could manage with less shark cartilage. I took seventy-five grams for two months, then fifty grams for six months. On July 9, 1996, I dropped to thirty-six grams for two months and dropped to thirty grams on September 9, 1996. On February 3, 1997, I increased my dose back up to fifty grams because Dr. Ruccio felt more comfortable if I did so. As long as my MRIs are good, I will continue to lower my dose until I reach twenty-four grams. This will be a slow weaning process. I think I'll stay at twenty-four grams as a maintenance dose. Being able to stay this long on shark cartilage is a major accomplishment in and of itself due to the bad taste. If you prepare the cartilage the way I did, you might find it more tolerable.

I prepared it in fresh juices. I believe very much in drinking live cells that are extracted from fresh fruits and vegetables. They say that cells stay alive for two hours after juicing; after that they will not be beneficial to you. You will need a good juicer, a blender, and an orange juice extractor. I try to juice four ounces of carrots accompanied by a combination of apples, oranges, grapes, spinach, celery, cabbage, beets, or any combination you like. I targeted specific organs I wanted to cleanse. You can find many recipes in the book *Raw Vegetable*

Juices by N. W. Walker, DSc. For example, I made shark cartilage with carrots, beets, and cucumbers at least once a day, targeting my gallstones.

I drank carrots and spinach to help normal regeneration of blood and for increasing oxygen transmission in the bloodstream. The combination I found most tolerable was carrots with apples, oranges, or grapes. After you've chosen the fresh organic (if possible) fruits and vegetables, you must juice approximately eight ounces. Once this is done, then put it in the blender along with whatever dose of shark cartilage you were recommended and mix it at a low speed for twenty to thirty seconds. Then pour it into a glass and continuously stir and drink, until finished. If you let it sit without stirring, it will turn into a paste that is not too appetizing. I find it helpful to hold my breath when drinking. Wash your equipment and put them away for the next treatment.

Shark cartilage can also be given through enemas if one cannot tolerate the taste. I strongly recommend everyone read the book *Sharks Don't Get Cancer* and the new book, *Sharks Still Don't Get Cancer*. In the book, it states that, unlike chemotherapy, shark cartilage is completely nontoxic and has no adverse side effects. Logically, if the blood networks can be kept from forming, then cancer growth can be prevented, which suggests that shark cartilage might be used not only as a therapy but also as a preventative or prophylactic measure. Shark cartilage has a track record of working very well with brain tumors, and that was a big plus for me. Doses should be spread out throughout the day. With shark cartilage, you must not eat anything one hour before and one hour after to allow the cartilage to absorb without competing with your food.

Next, I'll share a chart of my entire regimen, and how many times a day I took each herb and supplement in a single week.

Example of Early Treatment

x = times per day

EMPTY STOMACH	12-7	12-8	12-9	12-10	12-11	12-12	12-13
Echinacea	2x	2x	2x	2x	2x	2x	2x
Vital Veggies	2x	2x	2x	2x	2x	2x	2x
Earth Source Greens & More	2x	2x	2x	2x	2x	2x	2x
Cat's Claw	2x	2x	2x	2x	2x	2x	2x
Immunofin	2x	2x	2x	2x	2x	2x	2x
Ester-C w/ Bioflavonoids	2x	2x	2x	2x	2x	2x	2x
Phytaid	2x	2x	2x	2x	2x	2x	2x
Shark Cartilage	3x	3x	3x	3x	3x	3x	3x

WITH MEALS	12-7	12-8	12-9	12-10	12-11	12-12	12-13
Flaxseed Oil	1x	1x	1x	1x	1x	1x	1x
Astragulus	2x	2x	2x	2x	2x	2x	2x
CoQ-10 120mg	1x	1x	1x	1x	1x	1x	1x
Advanced Antioxidant Formula	2x	2x	2x	2x	2x	2x	2x
Daily Multi-vitamin	1x	1x	1x	1x	1x	1x	1x
Recovery Powder	1x	1x	1x	1x	1x	1x	1x
Myrrh-Goldenseal Plus	1x	1x	1x	1x	1x	1x	1x

MEDICATIONS	12-7	12-8	12-9	12-10	12-11	12-12	12-13
Phenytoin (anti-seizure)	2x	2x	2x	2x	2x	2x	2x
Dexamethasone (corticosteroid)	1x	2x	2x				
Ranitidine (stomach acid blocker)	1x	2x	2x				

I was going full steam ahead with all of my own added herbs. Anything that was good for the brain, circulation, liver, or my high cholesterol levels, I added. I constantly monitored my blood-work. I made sure everything was within normal levels. I did an ultrasound of all my internal organs to be sure they were working fine. I did discover that I had gallstones. I decided not to worry about them until I was well on my way to recovery. I planned to do a liver flush to rid myself of all those stones.

You can find an index of all the herbs and supplements I used, as well as their components and my comments on their use, at the back of this book.

When planning out a regimen of supplements, herbs, and med-ications, remember to spread out the pills during the day. Taking them too close together may decrease their effectiveness. Try not to take any medications within an hour of your herbs. This was a mistake I made in the beginning.

The experts could argue that for many vitamins and minerals, I doubled and tripled the necessary amount. I agree. I didn't know what I was doing in the beginning and mostly relied on my in-stincts and gut feelings at the time. This is all the guidance I had and the faith that it was God who was guiding me. Maybe I took too much of this and not enough of that, but I know one thing, I'm alive when I shouldn't be.

I've been told that my treatment is too difficult to understand and follow. I did what worked for me and my body while moni-toring my bloodwork regularly. I've been told that my method is too inconvenient, and my doctors have never heard of anything I was doing. Granted, it is very difficult to maintain good records and document every little thing. It's inconvenient because you must constantly be taking pills all day and you can't travel as much without lugging along with a juicer and blender. I know that chemotherapy and radiation treatments are short in comparison, but so is your life expectancy even with those conventional treatments.

What you must ask yourself is, "How badly do I want to live?"

There's a saying that nothing good in life comes easy, but I believe if you have something to live for and you want to live badly enough, you will try anything.

⚜ 12 ⚜

Divine Intervention

On January 27, 1996, I woke up feeling great. Elizabeth even let me sleep in a little longer. She dropped off Jimmy Jr. at the park for baseball and returned to pick me up. I was dropped off at his game and my wife went to take my daughter to her game. As I sat in the stands, I began to feel very bad inside. Immediately, I knew something was wrong. I was losing muscle control on the left side of my face. I wanted to leave, but I didn't want my youngest son, Jason, who was with me, to think there was something wrong. I waited a few minutes for Jimmy Jr. to finish his game and I took them both to Elizabeth. I began twitching a little, what they call Jacksonian seizures. I told Elizabeth to call my brother and have him pick me up and take me to a local hospital emergency room.

My brother Lazaro was flying through traffic and I was short of breath all the way. When we finally got there, I was stumbling to the door just to find them closed. I banged on the doors so they would open them. I did not get the reception I had pictured on the way over. "Yes, may I help you?" a nurse said very sarcastically.

I said, "I'm about to pass out, I can't breathe, I'm having seizures."

Her response shocked me. "Well, you'll have to walk down that hallway to the triage nurse out in the waiting area."

I said, "You want me to walk way down there when I can barely stand? Okay, okay, don't worry, that's a good lawsuit." I told the triage nurse my symptoms and they put me on a cot in the hallway. I began feeling worse by the minute. I asked my brother to call my wife, who was still in the park. He went out in the waiting area only to find all the phones in use. When he tried to come back in to find a phone, he was confronted by the security guard.

"Where do you think you're going?" he said.

"I have to find a phone because my brother's very sick."

"Oh no, I'm the chief of security and I say you can't go in."

At this point I heard my younger brother scream, "My brother is dying in there!" And he ran through the doors with the security in hot pursuit. Lazaro was very scared, especially since the doctors had said I only had three months to live, and three months had passed.

I saw the security guard calling on his walkie-talkie for backup. When security couldn't find him, he came back down the hallway in my direction. I stopped him and asked him to please leave my brother alone. I told him my brother was excited and he was the only family member I had there. That I wanted him by my side, so please don't bother him.

"No, I'm the chief of security, and no one talks to me like that!"

I said, "You don't know what is going on."

"Oh, yes, I know," he replied.

"No, you don't!"

"Oh, yes I do!"

"No, you don't!"

I was getting angry. He said, "I'm not even going to talk to you no more."

I may have threatened to kick the ever-loving shit out of him with my dying breath, but he said I was in no condition to do that anyway and left. When he was gone, Lazaro finally found his way back into the room.

I was unable to get out of the stretcher and both my arms became numb. I felt a seizure coming on and asked my brother to give me some of my Dilantin, which I had brought along with me.

"If I wait for them to see me, I'll have a seizure right here in the hallway," I said to my brother. The receptionist came to get my insurance card and have me sign three documents that I had no way of reading or understanding at that moment. My hands were shaking and numb. After I signed the first one, she told me there were two more. I couldn't believe that this was more important than finding out what was happening to me. I told her I couldn't sign any more.

She wanted my brother to sign and I said absolutely not. This is a trick they use to make someone else responsible for your bill if you can't pay it. So I scribbled my signature. My brother said, "Now that you have his money, do you think someone could attend to him?"

Someone came to talk to me and said he was the supervisor of I-don't-know-what and he wanted to know why I was so upset. He said I was level two—whatever that means—and I'd be attended to soon.

Finally, I was taken to a room and left there. Meanwhile, I'm short of breath. I asked my brother to look in the drawers for an oxygen mask and a humidifier. I'd worked in this emergency room and knew where everything was. I told him to put it up to eight liters, giving me approximately forty-five percent oxygen. At that moment the nurse walked in, and before she could ask what he was doing, I told her that I was the one who put on the mask. I was two to three steps ahead of them. I knew what they were going to say, do, and think before they even thought of it. The nurse asked me why I was using oxygen if my O_2 saturation was at one hundred percent. I told her that doesn't mean anything.

I asked her, "If a patient comes in with respiratory failure, wouldn't you give him oxygen?" She answered yes. "How do you know I'm not in respiratory failure if you haven't even asked for blood gas yet? My O_2 saturation may be one hundred percent simply because I'm hyperventilating."

I had the oxygen on for about ten minutes and I began to feel

71

much better. The doctor asked me to take it off to do a blood gas on room air and I agreed. A blood gas is when they remove blood from your artery and analyze it. This procedure is a good indicator of lung and kidney function and oxygenation of the blood. It is usually done in emergency situations. It also determines whether one is in an acidic or alkalotic state. This is very important in determining what will be the proper course of action.

It was a chess buddy of mine, John, that came to do my gas. He was in shock to see me. He gave me a look of being both happy and sad to see me. I hadn't seen him since my surgery three months previous.

While he did my gas, we talked about the good old times when me, him, and Art, another friend, played chess at work and got in all sorts of trouble because of it. He did an otherwise painful procedure with the professional skill I always knew he had. I didn't feel a thing. I asked him to bring me back the results because I felt if I didn't treat myself it wasn't going to get done.

John returned with my results, and as I suspected, I was hyperventilating. I had pH 7.56, CO_2 24. I was blowing off too much CO_2 (carbon dioxide). In a normal blood gas, the pH should be in the range of 7.35 to 7.45; anything higher than that would be considered alkalosis and anything below that would be acidic. The normal CO_2 should be in the range of 38 to 42. Anything higher than that would be acidic and anything lower would be considered alkalosis. This is what they call respiratory alkalosis. If the CO_2 is off, then it is a problem with the lungs. If the CO_2 is alkalosis and it matches the pH, which is also alkalosis, then this is respiratory alkalosis. My sodium bicarb and BE (base excess) was normal, meaning my kidneys were not involved. I knew if I didn't control this, eventually, I would tire out and just the opposite would occur. I would go into an acidic state—what they call respiratory acidosis—and eventually end up in respiratory failure.

I asked my brother Lazaro to put my simple mask at two liters and I put it over my face, covering the two holes on the side of the mask. Normally, a simple mask should be placed on five to ten liters because you need to blow off CO_2 accumulation from the mask.

At this point, the nurse walked in and asked what I was doing. I asked her, "Do you know what my blood gas results were?"

She said, "No."

I told her, "Well, I do. My CO_2 is twenty-four (normal being forty). I'm trying to rebreathe some of my own CO_2 to bring it back to normal."

She looked at me like I was crazy. At this point, they all thought I was nuts. The nurse needed to put in a heparin lock to get blood. She messed up on my left hand and blew up a vein. I was nice to her and told her to try the other hand, which she did okay. They had some bloodwork sent to the lab. They took a urine sample.

The emergency room physician walked in to ask me some questions about my medical history. I told him about my brain tumor and surgery and that I had refused all conventional radiation and chemotherapy. Once he knew that I refused all treatment, their attitude became, *Well, we can't do anything for him.* He told me that he was going to order a CAT scan of the brain and some lab work and chest x-rays. I told him that a CAT scan was not good enough to tell what was going on. I suggested an MRI instead. He said the CAT scan was sufficient.

I asked him, knowing the answer to my own question, "Can you tell if there is edema in the brain from the CAT scan?"

He said, "No."

"I didn't think so," I replied. I went on to express my concerns that maybe there was edema causing pressure in certain parts of the brain, giving me my current symptoms.

He said, "We don't do MRIs in the emergency room."

I didn't say any more even though I knew I could push. I could have argued by telling him the MRI machines were just down the hall from the ER.

I felt like telling him, "Let's skip all the politics of the hospital and get done what is needed for the patients." They came to do an x-ray and an EKG. They came to get me for the CAT scan. My wife, Elizabeth, was with me by this point, and I asked her to go home and get my phonebook because I didn't know what was going to happen and there were some people I wanted to see before things got worse. Among them were Joe and Linda Ligon, who had given me spiritual guidance. When I arrived at the CAT scan, I began to feel really bad. I was twitching more, dizzy, and urinating frequently.

When they put me on the table I said to the tech, "I don't think this is a good idea right now, because I'm twitching more and I'm afraid I'll have a seizure during the procedure."

They told me it was a short procedure. I asked if at least I could have some oxygen during the test. The tech called the doctor at the front desk and his response was no oxygen. I said, "What? He doesn't know what I need. Let me talk to him." I pleaded with the technician. He didn't even so much as acknowledge my presence; he just ignored me like I was a dog. His assistant taped my head down and put a strap around my arms like a straitjacket. I have witnessed this kind of treatment of patients many times in my professional career. I never approved of it then and I definitely didn't like it done to me. It's the most degrading thing one human can do to another.

My twitches were getting worse throughout the whole procedure. The only thing I could do was pray that God would be with me and see me through this ordeal. It is an absolute crime what some healthcare providers do to patients behind closed doors.

This reminded me of a patient I once cared for early on in my career. He was a very nice man with a beautiful family who was unfortunate enough to have very bad asthma. I had to do bronchodilator treatment with albuterol every two hours to keep his lungs open. During the middle of the night, I went to give him his treatment and I found the room full of nurses and the resident making a big commotion around the patient. I had a close friend with me whom I was orienting to the hospital. He was a new employee and a former teacher and mentor of mine. The doctor was talking to the patient about intubating him (placing a tube in his lungs to breathe) and putting him on a life support ventilator.

He had no clue as to what the doctor was telling him, and, like the average person who doesn't know, he put his faith in the resident. Like most patients, one thinks that it's for his own good, but what he didn't know was that once you go on a ventilator, it's not so easy to get off. The rumor was he wanted to practice his intubation technique, but I don't know if that was true or not. Seeing what was occurring, I spoke to the resident and told him that I was very familiar with this patient and all that he needed was an aerosol treatment and he would be okay. He had been like that before and twenty minutes after the treatments he was fine.

His response was, "*I AM THE DOCTOR* and I say we intubate, so prepare the tube and get a ventilator." The intubation began, and I will never forget the fear in the patient's eyes. The resident stuck the tube in the esophagus instead of the trachea. "Okay, pull the tube and I'll try again." So he tried again, and again, missing every time.

It was beginning to look like a bloody mess with all the trauma to the throat area. Finally, after the fourth or fifth attempt, the resident was frustrated and he said, "There, it's in." I looked at my partner and we both looked at the patient's stomach. Every time I gave a breath with the bag valve mask, the patient's stomach would rise higher and higher.

I said, "Doc, look at the patient's stomach. We are ventilating his stomach, not his lungs."

"I'm the doctor here and I say it's in! Besides, look at his chest, it's rising."

My partner told me to remove the bag valve mask and he pushed on his stomach and all this air was expelled out. "Oh yes, it's all right," my partner said.

I told the doctor the only reason his chest was rising was because he was trying to breathe not only around his inflamed bronchial, but also this tube he had in his esophagus that was pressing against the trachea.

Again, he said that *he* was the doctor. "I want a blood gas and an x-ray. Call me if there are any more problems," he said.

I looked at my partner and the nurses and said, "I hope he doesn't go very far. This patient is going to code any minute." It took less than five minutes before the patient finally gave up breathing.

"CODE BLUE, TELEMETRY, CODE BLUE, TELEMETRY," the announcement sounded throughout the hospital.

Back came the resident screaming orders. "Get the crash cart! Lidocaine, epinephrine, sodium bicarbonate, blood gas." The code was long and throughout the code, me and my partner were telling him that if he didn't establish an airway, there was no way he going to make it.

"What are you talking about? The airway is established, he is intubated."

There was no way we could change his mind. He knew that he couldn't intubate this man and was too proud to admit it or ask someone else to try, even if it cost this patient his life. I felt like ripping the tube out and forcing him to intubate the patient. This option may not have been helpful because he probably couldn't reintubate. If I did that, I might have been blamed for his death if he didn't make it.

If I have learned anything working in hospitals, it is that doctors will always try to blame someone else for their mistakes. Respiratory therapists are commonly used scapegoats not only for doctors, but for nurses as well. Eventually, he went flatline.

"Charge the paddles," he commanded.

Shocking the patient is usually only effective when a patient is in ventricular fibrillation or atrial fibrillation. I've always seen them give lidocaine when a patient is flatline. He must have shocked this poor man at least ten times with no response. My partner and I were not surprised, but were powerless to do anything about it. This doctor didn't follow the ABCs. A for airway is the first thing one must establish. This was not done. Then

B for breathing, which wasn't possible because there was no airway. Finally, **C** for circulation. There's no sense in circulating blood if it's not carrying oxygen. So the bottom line is if you don't do **A**, don't bother with **B** and **C**.

Eventually, he passed away and the code was terminated. I said a prayer for this unfortunate soul that happened to fall into the hands of a savage beast. Things like this happen all the time behind closed doors. This is legal murder, and it happens every day in a hospital in this country. The family members are never allowed in the room to witness this butchery; that's why security is called in every Code Blue. They keep them away so that they don't see something that they might get sued for later. The hospital employees are afraid to speak out for fear they'll lose their much-needed jobs and be blackballed from every other area hospital. What really upset me the most was when I heard the resident speaking to the grieving family.

He said, "We tried everything we could, but he had a heart attack and his heart just gave out." If they only knew the truth. All the patient needed was a ten-minute breathing treatment and he would have been watching TV and enjoying his family.

This same doctor called me to the emergency room one night to do a blood gas on a patient with chronic obstructive pulmonary disease, or COPD. These patients normally retain carbon dioxide and are breathing on what we call their hypoxic drive. Hypoxic drive means stimulus to breathing due to lack of oxygen. This simply means the only reason these patients stay breathing is that their bodies sense a lack of oxygen. These patients cannot be given high concentrations of oxygen or they'll stop breathing. He orders me to put the patient on a simple mask at two liters.

Immediately, I began to question his decision, only to get his usual response: "I'm the doctor here!"

"Doctor, a simple mask delivers from thirty-five to fifty-five percent oxygen, and that is too much for a COPD patient," I told him.

"I know that, that is why I only want him on two liters of oxygen. I do know what I am doing," he responded.

I said to him, "Doctor, you cannot give two liters of oxygen with a simple mask. You must give at least five to ten liters to blow off excessive CO_2 buildup in the mask. You have to put him in a nasal cannula at one to two liters."

I couldn't believe this doctor was treating patients. This was simple, basic knowledge that any respiratory therapist knew in their first month of school.

"I'm the doctor here and I say two liters of simple mask!"

There was no sense in arguing with people like this who are on a constant ego trip. I went back to my unit thinking there would be another Code Blue in the emergency room soon. If a COPD patient who already has a CO_2 in the nineties (normal being forty) begins to rebreathe his accumulating CO_2 in the mask, he will go into respiratory failure for sure. Luckily for this man, I saw the patient's pulmonologist, who was doing his rounds in the unit. I told him, "By the way, I just saw one of your patients in the emergency room. His CO_2 was in the nineties and I put him on a simple mask at two liters."

"What did you say?"

"Oh yes, I tried to explain it to the emergency physician, and he told me he was the doctor so I left."

He picked up the phone and really let that guy have it. He ordered the resident to put him on a nasal cannula at two liters just like I told him. He didn't speak to me for at least six months.

There may be a doctor like this in your emergency room. There are some good ones, but the bad ones are responsible for destroying people's confidence. When one has witnessed events like this, it's no wonder you lose your faith in doctors fast. That's why I was so upset in the emergency room. My friend Henry would say to me, "Jimmy, don't get so upset, it's not good for you."

I said, "I'm not upset so much for myself, because at least I can defend myself. What about the twenty or so other people in this emergency room that don't know what's going on and don't know how to defend themselves? This abuse must end! The hospitals are more at fault than the healthcare providers. They are the hypocrites that advertise how much they care about the quality and the welfare of the patients. The translation of that propaganda is, we want to treat more patients with less staff. That way the net profits are more. Less staff spells out more cash."

After the CAT scan, I was taken back to my room. I grabbed the oxygen mask and I felt a little better. They only allowed one person in to see me at a time. When one would leave, I felt very alone.

That's when it happened.

I saw Jesus in the corner of the ceiling, and this amazing warmth surrounded my body. I said, "Thank you, Lord, for being here for me." I didn't know if that was a good or bad sign, but I did feel more at ease. As time passed, I began to lose strength and movement on my left side. The doctor and nurses thought I was making it all up.

They really believed that I was crazy. I must have brain damage because of my tumor. They asked my wife, Elizabeth, "Has he been depressed lately? I understand he has a very serious terminal illness."

"No, on the contrary, he's been very outgoing and happy and spending a lot of time with his three kids. This is the first time since surgery that he's had seizures," Elizabeth told them. Oh well, there goes that theory. They expected a different response.

Meanwhile, back in the room, I had seen Jesus two more times in the corner of the ceiling, only appearing when I was alone. I was getting worse by the moment. I was now unable to move any part of my body and had very labored breathing. The doctor finally walked in. I had been asking for him for a very long time and he never came. I guess terminal patients that refuse conventional treatment are not a priority.

He was looking at his test results and told me with a straight face, "Well, Jimmy, we don't seem to find anything eminently wrong with you. Your CAT scan shows that your intracranial pressures are fine."

"What did you say?" I asked. "How could you possibly know what my intracranial pressures are from a CAT scan? The only way you can know that is if you insert a tube into my head and connect it to an intracranial monitor," I said to him.

His response was, "Do you want me to put one in?" in a very sarcastic and disrespectful way.

I said, "No, just don't be telling me something that you know is not accurate and you have no way of knowing."

"You seem to be fine," he said.

"Let me ask you a question, Doctor. If you've done all your tests, have all your results, and your professional opinion is that I'm okay, then why is it that I'm lying here unable to move and twitching all over?"

He replied, "Well, I'm only an ER physician and I don't know your history."

I said, "Yes, you are the ER physician, and I am a patient in the ER, and whatever decision you make is going to affect me."

He said, "What is it that you are concerned about?"

"I know what your intentions are; you want to discharge me and send me home, so I could have a seizure in front of my kids, and by the time fire rescue comes and brings me back I'll be dead. If you want me to leave, you're going to have to carry me, because I can't move. I think you should at least admit me for twenty-four-hour observation," I told him.

While trying his best to terminate the conversation, he made his exit, saying, "Yeah, yeah," his eyes never making contact with mine.

I knew I didn't have much time. I didn't want my younger brother to see me like this and I couldn't even open my eyes anymore. That's when I remembered what my minister had said in one of his sermons. He talked about how Jesus healed the sick when he was on earth. He never refused anyone, and some days he would heal hundreds at a time, taking on all their illness onto himself. Can you imagine the pain he went through?

I wanted to tell my lifelong friend Henry a story; it was probably the last one I would tell. I told him about a woman who was the mother of Elizabeth's friend, who also had a brain tumor. She had gone through all the conventional treatments. Radiation, chemotherapy, and the gamma knife twice. The last gamma knife left her paralyzed on the left side. With all her insurance money gone, they sent her home to die. For three weeks she wouldn't wake up except to be fed. The only time she spoke was to ask that I go see her.

Before she and I were sick, we didn't even know each other, so I was surprised at her request. Of course, I went to see her fully armed with all the knowledge I had acquired during my three months of research into alternative therapies, including what seemed to be working for me. The first thing I did was to ask to be left alone with her for a moment. I knew that God was the one who was really going to save her and me. I called her name.

"Lucy, can you hear me?" She nodded her head yes. "Are you still breathing?" I asked her.

She answered me in very labored breathing, "Yes."

Her hand tightly squeezed my own. I told her that as long as she was breathing she still had a chance; only God could tell her when her time was up. "Lucy, I have the Lord with me, and He is going to heal you."

I said a special prayer. I pleaded with God to find it in his heart to bring this woman back to health. Afterward I talked to her daughter and spent a couple of hours going over all the herbs I was taking and what they were good for. In my heart, I knew they wouldn't give it to her and only God could save her. I had complete faith that He would.

I told Henry the story briefly, and the reason I felt it was significant was that I had been fine until three days after I went to Lucy's house. I told Henry of what Jesus did in taking on others' illnesses, and if this was the mission God had for me, to take on others' illnesses, that was fine with me. I would go through the suffering a thousand times if that's what the Lord wished.

"I just hope, Lord, that at the same time you're taking me, that you're healing Lucy," I said to the Lord.

I was very close to the end now. I knew it because I was agonal breathing. This is the way people breathe when they are taking their last breaths. They're short and shallow breaths with long pauses in between. I'd seen it many times during my career. It's true that your hearing is the last to go, because I was very aware of everything that was happening around me. The nurses had come in to take my pressure and see what was going on.

That's when I remembered another sermon the minister had given us. He told us a hypothetical story of a man hanging on a branch off the side of a cliff. He called out, "Help! Someone help me!"

The Lord answered, "Yes, I hear you. What can I do for you?"

"Save me, get me out of this mess!" the man cried.

"Okay, I'll save you, just let go," the Lord replied.

After a long pause, the man said, "Is there anyone else out there?" He had no faith.

I was already at the point where I said to myself, "Okay, Lord, I'm letting go of that branch, so catch me in Your arms. I surrender myself to You."

At that exact moment, I began to feel breaths being forced into my lungs just like a 7200 ventilator would do when giving manual sighs. Each breath was deeper and deeper than the previous. With each breath, I felt my legs rise higher and higher as if someone were picking them up, but I didn't feel any hands. It was the same sensation that one would feel when your legs float up in water.

All of a sudden, I began to feel like I could just jump out of the bed. Something was telling me that is exactly what I had to do and give the Lord all the credit. After I had exhaled that fourth and deepest breath of all, I had an amazing burst of energy and jumped right up onto the edge of the bed. The nurses were in shock because moments earlier I was completely paralyzed and posturing.

That happens just before someone dies. It means your hands,

arms, and feet turn in all weird directions. My friend Henry told me to lie back down. I looked him straight in the eyes and told him, "Henry, you don't understand. I've seen the Lord three times in this room and He wants me to get up and walk out of here."

I picked up all my clothes, dressed, and met Elizabeth in front of the nurse's station. Seconds earlier she was on the phone in the lobby talking to my brother, who told her to hurry to the room. So she was in shock to see me walking in the ER.

I told the doctor that the best doctor in the world had healed me, and that was God. Everyone in the emergency room really thought I was crazy now. I put my shoes on in front of the door, and with a heparin lock still on, I walked out looking for my van. My friend Henry asked me if I was sure that I was okay, because I was stumbling a little.

"Do you want to race to the car?" I asked him.

I also saw great relief in my younger brother's eyes; he was really stressed throughout this whole ordeal. We were always very close. I'm sixteen years older than him, and ever since he was a baby I would always take him everywhere I went.

My wife and I boarded our van and I said, "Let's get out of here before they finish me off." But, before we reached the main street, I said to Elizabeth, "We better go back and sign out, or else the insurance company won't pay the emergency room bill." I walked back to the ER and the doctor said he had just spoken with my oncologist and he wanted to call him back, and asked if I could wait in the room that I was in. I said, "I'll wait out in the waiting room better. I'm sure there are people out there waiting who really need a bed a lot more than I do, give it to them."

So I went out to the waiting room area and decided to practice what I preach. I've said in the past, "Abuse no one, and if you are abused, pray for your abuser." I went straight to the security guard who gave me and my brother a hard time and shook his hand. "I just want to apologize for the hard time we gave you, but things were really bad in there for me. I saw the Lord and He saved me. It's not good to have enemies; we are all in this together, and what one does affects us all. By the way, don't I know you? You look very familiar."

It turned out that we knew each other from the years I worked in that hospital. He didn't recognize me because I had lost thirty-five pounds. I was called back to sign out and pick up some papers, and that was that. My younger brother was very relieved and much happier now.

Throughout this whole ordeal, I was saying to myself, *If I could only go to the bathroom, I would feel better.* When I arrived at home, I found what appeared to be thousands of parasites in my stool.

They appeared similar to the pictures shown in the book *The Cure for All Cancers.* I spent the next three days passing these apparent parasites.

13

The Skeptics

O nce I began talking about my success, all the skeptics came out of the woodworks. The doctors couldn't explain the reason why my tumor was not growing. At the same time, they refused to accept the possibility that it might have been because of shark cartilage. One radiologist said that I must have been misdiagnosed. I explained that I had four opinions and DNA analysis to prove that it wasn't a misdiagnosis.

Their argument is they know many people who have taken shark cartilage and it's only helped a few, and most people have not benefited from the use of shark cartilage at all. My response to that is, I know of some people whom it hasn't helped also. In my opinion, they didn't administer the shark cartilage properly or use the right product or dosages. Also, my success was not a result of shark cartilage alone. I believe my many other herbs, supplements, and faith all were important contributors.

I am not surprised by all the skeptics, because I know what I did is not mainstream and it is very hard to swim upstream. I believe that shark cartilage could help more people if it were taken more seriously and more studies were conducted.

I wish more people had an open mind. If an all-natural protocol were developed and proven, I am positive that the clear majority would choose it rather than a toxic treatment. When the skeptics hear of someone who has done something different and has succeeded, it is always brushed aside as a fluke.

In my opinion, it's not a fluke. I happen to be a very concerned person who is outraged by the medical establishment for not being serious about finding a cure for brain cancer. I worked in the medical field for twelve years and knew nothing about alternatives.

When the medical doctors wrote me off as a statistic, I got angry. I am not a statistic! I am a living, breathing human being just like they are. I had a family, friends, and a career. I was not ready to die. I searched for hope and found it with supplements and faith. What's wrong with that?

I am sorry it is not proven science. I'm sorry they don't believe in it. That is their problem, not mine. Who cares if it is not endorsed by the greatest medical minds of our time? History may look back at today as barbaric times when we tortured our own people all in the name of medicine.

I didn't have time to wait for the future or for some red tape to be sorted out. I was desperate in the same manner hundreds of thousands of people are right now. People are suffering from cancer and are fighting with the clock.

I am only one voice screaming in the darkness. I doubt anyone will hear me. The more people I can reach with the truth, the more screaming voices there will be. Eventually, with enough people screaming, someone will listen.

As long as I have breath in my lungs, I will try to help cancer patients and bring them hope! It's been argued that shark cartilage has only helped a few, but for the vast majority, it didn't. Well, I could argue the same about radiation and chemotherapy as a treatment for glioblastoma multiforme.

It has helped a very few live a little longer in agony, but the vast majority are dead. I ask you, what is the difference between the two treatments except for cost? Chemotherapy and radiation could easily run into the hundreds of thousands of dollars, while shark cartilage may run between eight to ten thousand dollars a year. So how could they argue that one should not take shark cartilage if the treatment they offer, in my opinion, is worthless?

By their own admission, it will not cure you. So what should a person in my situation do, just sit back and wait to die? I don't think so!

I feel terrible when I have to tell someone that has already endured the pain of these treatments that they are not necessary.

It has been argued that shark cartilage is all a scam, and some people don't like the way it is marketed. I am not saying that there aren't scam artists out there trying to make a fast buck. There are. I was almost a victim of one of those scams. When I first went looking for the shark cartilage in the health food store, I was sold worthless injectables. Many people are victims of these criminals. Owners of health food stores many times pass themselves off as experts and are far from it. Many don't know anything.

I believe this is one of the reasons for the bad publicity and failures people experience with shark cartilage. This is why I am in favor of organized and well-structured studies with shark cartilage.

I am one person, and I had one successful remission. That's one hundred percent in my book. Since I'm talking about percentages, here are some interesting statistics. Radiation and chemotherapy have a zero percent success rate in curing glioblastoma multiforme brain tumors, but are approved by the FDA and used as a standard treatment for glioblastoma multiforme.[16]

It's been argued that Dr. Lane is lining his pockets making millions selling shark cartilage. I don't know about that; it sounds a little steep. What they don't mention is that Dr. Lane has spent close to $250,000 of his own money to research shark cartilage because the government would not provide him with research grants. What doctor would believe in his own convictions enough to do that? I understand that he is making money, but isn't this the American way? How much are they making off chemotherapy

---

[16] Trifiletti, Daniel M., "Mayo Clinic Calls out Need for Aggressive Glioblastoma Treatment," *Forefront*, December 2019.
https://www.mayo.edu/research/forefront/mayo-clinic-calls-out-need-for-aggressive-glioblastoma-treatment.

and radiation treatments, and who is lining their pockets with that money?

No one talks about that, right? I have heard people argue that it's the placebo effect that helped the few obtain good results. What does this mean? I do not think this theory holds water. If anyone looks up my diagnosis—glioblastoma multiforme grade IV—they will find out that it is an extremely vicious malignant tumor for which there is no known effective treatment.

No matter how much anyone thinks they are going to get better, if you do not attack this cancer it will spread. I believe that positive thinking is important and a part of the overall treatment. By itself, I do not see it working, because this tumor grows too fast and it will kill you.

I have been told that my case was one in a million—a miracle. Yes, it was a miracle. But I think the reason I am one in a million is because only one in a million would bypass the medical establishment. Only one in a million may have the faith that I had in God and in nature.

If a million people did what I did, I would think there would be close to a million miracles. Whenever I am asked to visit a cancer patient, I tell them how important it is to believe in God and pray for Him to cure you. I also tell them to picture themselves drowning in the ocean. If you ask God to save you, God might say, "All right, I'll save you, here's a life preserver." Once the life preserver is thrown to you, it is up to you to grab it or drown.

Meaning, if you want to live, you have to make the effort. You have to take charge of your own health. Once the way is shown to you, the ball is in your court. You have to believe in what you're doing.

Be strong, be confident, and most importantly, have faith.

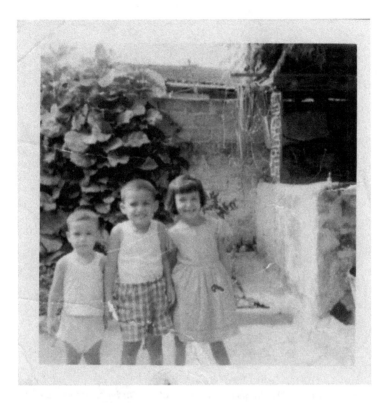

Jimmy (farthest left) and his two older siblings, Tony and Aida, standing in front of their home in Cuba in 1959.

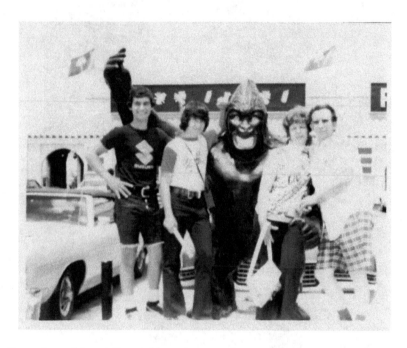

Jimmy (second from left) with his mother, Eva, father, Antonio, and brother Tony in New Jersey in 1972.

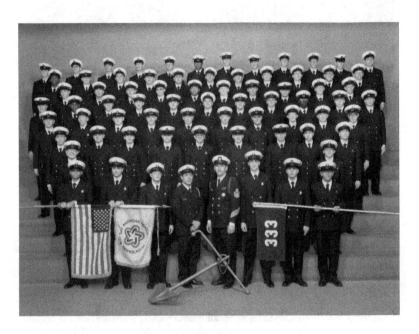

Jimmy's naval basic training graduation photo in 1974. He's in the second row, second from right.

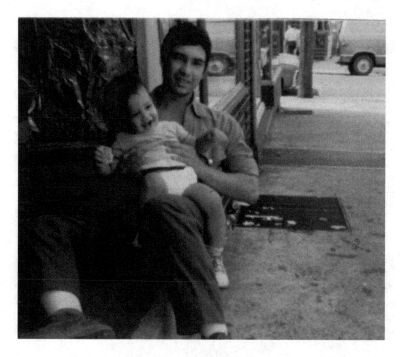

Jimmy on one of his trips home from the military with his little brother Lazaro outside their father's New Jersey flower shop in 1975.

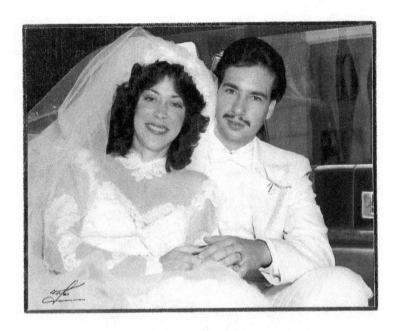

Jimmy marries his wife, Elizabeth, in 1983.

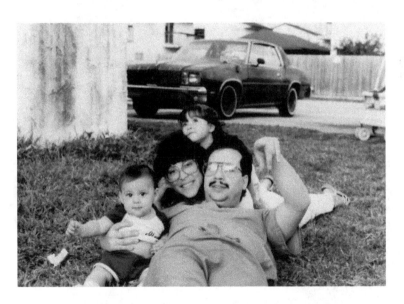

Jimmy with wife, Elizabeth, daughter, Jamie, and son Jimmy Jr. in front of their home in Miami in 1988.

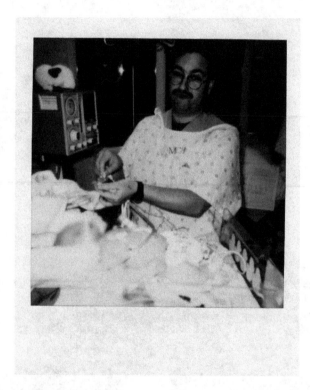

Jimmy in an undated photo at his job as a respiratory therapist in the NICU at Miami Children's Hospital.

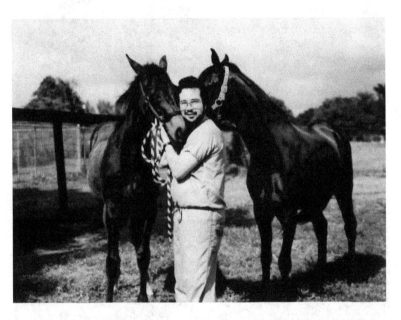

Jimmy loved horses and posed with his horse Bandango Slew, on the right, and one other horse in 1992.

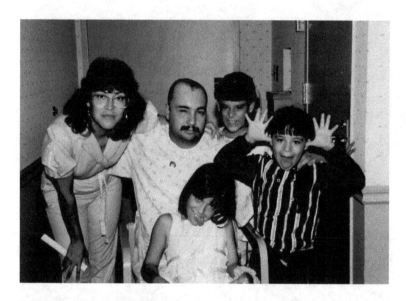

After his first seizure and first surgery to remove a golf ball–sized glioblastoma multiforme grade IV tumor from his brain in 1995, Jimmy poses with his wife and kids in the hospital.

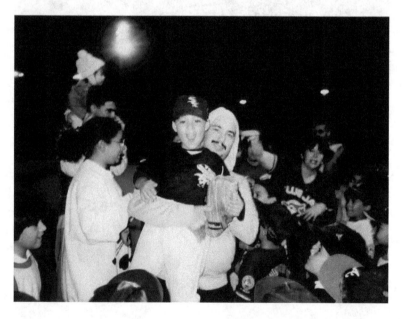

After returning home from his first surgery in 1995, Jimmy holds up his son Jason at a baseball game at Tamiami Park.

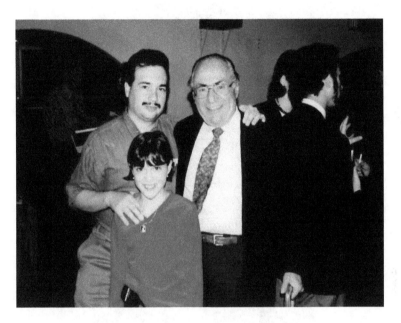

Jimmy poses with Dr. William Lane and daughter, Jamie (yes, I'm wearing a beeper), at a speech Dr. Lane was giving in Miami in 1996.

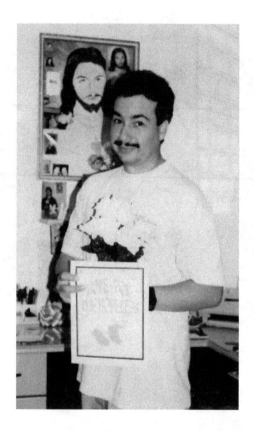

*Jimmy poses with the first cover of his book, Hope for the Hopeless, in 1997,
having already far outpaced his three-month life expectancy.*

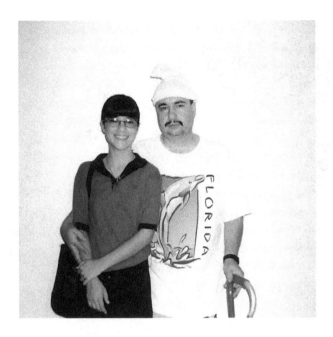

Jimmy and daughter, Jamie, posing at home after his second surgery to remove a recurrent glioblastoma multiforme grade IV tumor in 1998, about three years after this first surgery and diagnosis.

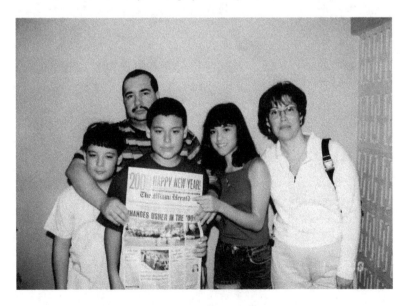

Jimmy and family holding a newspaper celebrating the year 2000.

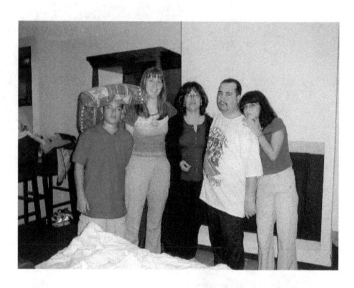

Jimmy in Los Angeles, California, in October 2000 the night before his third brain tumor removal surgery, posing with son Jimmy Jr.; sister-in-law Deanna; wife, Elizabeth; and daughter, Jamie

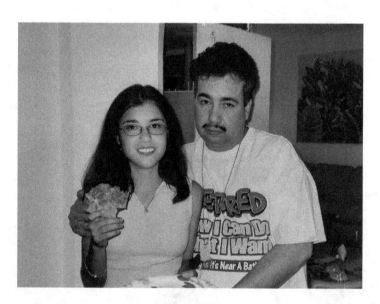

Jimmy with daughter, Jamie, on her fifteenth birthday in 2001. Around his neck, he wears a whistle and his anti-seizure medication.

✤ 14 ✤

Conversation with Dr. Dante Ruccio

After seventeen months of success, I called Dr. Dante Ruccio (who got his degree in naturopathic medicine from La Salle University in 1991) to let him know that I was writing a book. He was thrilled and was willing to assist me in writing this chapter. Here is our conversation.

DR. RUCCIO: If you would have listened to the medical profession and done the chemotherapy, it would not even have touched that brain tumor. Glioblastoma happens to be a very aggressive tumor, but they probably would have gone ahead with the chemotherapy because that's all they know. This is what the medical profession does. They have statistics. Based on statistics they know what works and what doesn't work. Therefore, if glioblastoma is untreatable with chemotherapy, the question is, why do they use it?

Is it a monetary thing? Is it a business decision? In my opinion, that's what I think it is. In many cases, I have CAT scans and MRIs here where people have failed on chemotherapy and then went on to do the same therapy you decided to use.

When they do get a response, they'll tell you it was the chemotherapy even though the chemotherapy was interrupted two years ago. I do not believe this is science, but they are in control of the science. They could do what they want, and I believe it's to keep the pharmaceutical companies going and keep this whole monopoly and industry alive. I don't believe that any medical doctor should have the right to set standards on a subject that they are not trained in, nor do they have a degree in. I believe, politically, politicians who pass laws in their favor forget that they could come down with cancer. They could come down with many degenerative diseases and the only options and treatments are going to be toxic molecular-restructured chemicals which do not assimilate nor identify with your own body chemistry. Many medical doctors understand this. There is a very articulate doctor from the University of Arizona that stated this on public television. All of a sudden, when he was talking about chemotherapy, indicating that when we look back we are going to even wonder why we did this to people, he got cut off.

JIMMY: Really?

DR. RUCCIO: They had cut the TV program right off. What's going on in this field is that the medical profession calls drugs medicine and natural remedies drugs. The fact of the matter is if anyone advises and gives an opinion which cures someone, in my opinion, that is the practice of medicine. Even if I tell you to eat a carrot and it will make your eyes better. I don't believe that jurisdictions should come under their category, because none of them are trained in the field of alternatives.

The whole thing, in a nutshell, is this: In this country, we have been doing medicine for about two hundred years. We have the best diagnostics in the world and we cure nothing.

In Europe, they've been practicing medicine for thousands of years, yet they [American doctors] never accept any studies from Europe, and only their studies count. Like they are the gods in the field. I personally believe that the public needs to call their senators in Washington and state legislators. Start a whole different system where naturopathic physicians and naturopathic consultants practice the field that they were trained in without being intimidated by the medical profession.

For instance, a naturopathic physician has to go in front of a medical board. I don't think there should be a medical board; I think there should be a naturopathic board.*

It's like going to a kangaroo court. I don't believe that the prosecutors in the various states have the right to raid alternative doctors, specifically because they don't have any knowledge about anything. Even if I could prove patients have been turned around, that information falls on deaf ears.

I'll give you an example of how they are covering things up. There is one girl down by Florida who had two brain tumors, one that has disappeared. I have the radiological report here. The radiologist put down that the tumor has disappeared from a surgical procedure. This person never had surgery.

There is also a little girl in New Mexico with a brain tumor who is two years old.

The doctors terrorized the mom into using chemotherapy even though she didn't want to use it. By the way, as you know, I don't oppose surgery. If you have

---

* There are now the North American Board of Naturopathic Examiners (NABNE) and the American Association of Naturopathic Physicians (AANP).

to remove the tumor, I think the surgeons do a good job. In this particular case, the surgeon said that the only way he would follow the case is if she did the surgery. Which is okay, and she had previous surgery and it grew back, but they had to do chemotherapy. I just talked with the person yesterday, and already the child's blood count is going down and various other complications are starting to set in. Now, this baby has enough trouble as it is, let alone with conventional medicine causing complications that didn't exist before.

This is what's wrong. There are 320,000 deaths a year from drug overuse in hospitals. There are many cancer patients that expire and they'll put down on the death certificate that they died from heart failure. Well, of course, but the primary cause is either cancer or the treatment or starvation. If a person dies and he has cancer, the cause should indicate that it was cancer. Therefore, the statistics are lower than what they really are.

JIMMY: You're right about that. Just recently Senator Paul Tsongas died. Everyone knows he has been fighting cancer for many years, and they said he died of pneumonia.

DR. RUCCIO: If you survive breast cancer for five years, they are calling this a cure. Well, to me, a cure is a cure is a cure. If you come back with metastasis to the liver, which is the same type of tumor of the breast cancer cell, or that type of neoplasm— that is not a cure.

Many of the people who have chemotherapy after surgery are made to think that the chemotherapy has caused tumor markers to go down. The fact is, it was reduced due to the removal of the tumor. When you remove a tumor automatically, the tumor markers will read lower than what they were. They put these people on chemotherapy for six months, five months, a year, whatever, and they will never take a CAT scan until they are finished with the chemotherapy. The reason that they won't take a CAT scan in between the chemotherapy is that if they had to come back and tell the patient that the tumor is still growing, most people will ask, why am I taking the chemotherapy? As long as they can milk the insurance company, they are going to keep doing it. As you know, Jimmy, I never took a dime from you. I don't take money from anyone.

If anyone wants to talk about people being charlatans, well then, maybe we could put some of the medical profession — not all — in that category. I think this whole thing has to be exposed. People have to understand that practically every drug that a pharmaceutical company produces has consequences. They take drugs for prostate cancer that cause liver problems, they're giving women tamoxifen, which may open them up to cancer of the uterine cervix later on. When you're taking chemotherapy, you are getting complications and problems you didn't have.

JIMMY Do you think that chemotherapy in some cases actually causes the deaths?

DR. RUCCIO: Yes, the only way I think chemotherapy works is on certain leukemia and some non–Hodgkin's disease. I don't believe they have any effect on hard tumors. I think they should put it on the record; they have a duty and obligation that when a person is on shark cartilage it should read in the radiological report, and then let the experts decide what is working and what is not working. But they just don't want this to happen.

JIMMY: I know I tried to convince the radiologist that reads my MRIs to document the fact that I was treated with shark cartilage. I didn't get very far; they just don't want to get involved. I asked if I were on radiation and chemotherapy if they would indicate that on the report under "History." They said yes, so I asked why, if I am being treated with shark cartilage successfully, it's not documented. I was unable to get a straight answer. As a consolation, they did state the fact that I had no history of chemotherapy and radiation.

This makes it look as though I didn't do anything, and that's not true. This may mislead others that read my MRI report later. I think they fear that if they document on a radiological report the fact that I was treated with shark cartilage, it will give it credibility. Why else would they refuse to document the truth?

DR. RUCCIO: First of all, another reason is that they are egomaniacs, many of them; they are egotistical, they suffer from tunnel vision, they are so brainwashed that it is pathetic. They cannot see anything any other way. They do not want to give any credit to other health professionals. If you would have listened to the doctors and done the treatment they wanted you to do, do you seriously think you would be here?

JIMMY: No, I think I would be dead.

DR. RUCCIO: You had one operation, is that correct?

JIMMY: One, that's it. I had some residue, but it hasn't grown back because of the shark cartilage.

DR. RUCCIO: The shark cartilage definitely helped, because people with glioblastomas all die. The prostate cancers are doing pretty good. The colon and liver do well. Adenocarcinoma of the lung does well. I have to be honest and reasonable, there is a point of no return, that no matter what you do it is not going to work. What doctors do too often is terrorize people into using chemotherapy. They give them a line that they will live longer if they do radiation and chemotherapy.

First of all, they perpetrated a fraud because, again, the medical profession knows and it is documented that chemotherapy does not penetrate the blood-brain barrier. I know some of them will ask how the shark cartilage gets through the blood-brain barrier.

First of all, shark cartilage is a food supplement, and all food is recognized by the brain and by the body as friendly material. Whatever nutrients are in the shark cartilage will be accepted by the brain as friendly material. The brain has a mechanism to protect it from toxic chemicals, and that is why these chemicals do not get in there. Again, I have to reemphasize, I don't want to be redundant, but if you could remove that tumor with surgery, you remove it. I also have some people that are inoperable and they're starting to get results. In brain tumors, sometimes there is edema and there is fluid. If you don't get the fluid out, the fluid will act the same as the brain tumor and put pressure on the brain. It will constrict the blood supply, causing a midline shift, which shifts the brain over and you can die from that.

JIMMY: How do you distinguish edema from cerebral spinal fluid?

DR. RUCCIO: Well, your physician did that. He identified that it was really spinal fluid. You always have spinal fluid kind of flowing in and out of the brain. At that particular time when I asked you to check that out and ask your physician, that was done more or less as a precaution. It's better to be safe than to be sorry. I thought that was the best advice that I could give you.

Ninety-nine percent of the people that I consult with definitely have to be also monitored by a physician. For blood tests, MRI, CAT scans, and so on and so forth. I have no qualms about that, but what I do resent is when a person goes into a doctor's office and they tell them they have three months to live when maybe they have three years. Nobody knows how long a person has to live when they have cancer. Unless it's throughout your whole body.

If it's the beginning and it's the primary and one centimeter, you're not dying. Unless it's some kind of freak situation that takes place.

As far as Dr. Lane, I think the man deserves a Nobel Prize for what he has brought to the world. Maybe someday they will be able to do something injectable. At this point, they are unable to do that.

The reason alternatives are catching on is because the American people today are smarter than they were forty or fifty years ago. They are taking charge of their own health. They are not listening to what one medical doctor may say; they are getting everyone's opinion. The medical establishment is not curing degenerative diseases like arthritis. They don't understand the first thing about vitamins. They do not know the difference between broccoli and a stone.

We studied antioxidants twenty years ago and now they are on television like they are the experts. There was a study done in Europe about beta carotene, and the study was flawed specifically because they used a synthetic form of beta carotene. When synthetic versus a natural beta carotene, like, say, extracted from a carrot or sweet potato, the natural beta carotene has cofactors that work synergistically together; that is the difference between natural and synthetics. They put it all over television, "Oh, beta carotene may increase your chance of getting lung cancer."

JIMMY: I heard about that.

DR. RUCCIO: That is a bunch of bolognas, because you cannot compare the response of a synthetic product versus a natural product.

JIMMY: They did not say it was a synthetic product.

DR. RUCCIO: They didn't say that. An eggplant has five hundred chemicals in it, and if you juiced an eggplant, and you put, let's say, two ounces of the juice and two ounces of the water and drank it three times a day, probably in ninety days, it will lower your cholesterol twenty percent. The pharmaceuticals took that, and they synthesized what they thought was the active ingredient, leaving the other four hundred ninety-nine chemicals behind, so it may not work the same and has side effects.

This is what goes on. They are not interested in natural remedies because they cannot patent them. They are also interested in trying to classify a natural remedy as a drug, because then it would come under their domain.

When this occurs, then you would have to go to a doctor and spend sixty, seventy, eighty, or ninety dollars, whatever they charge you for the visit, and he is going to give you a prescription for some stupid vitamin that is not even therapeutic.

The American public has to start waking itself up. No one beats the medical profession when it comes to a life-threatening situation. If your appendix bursts, or you get hit by a car, or you need a heart transplant or a liver transplant, or you need that type of thing, nobody is better than American medical doctors. When it comes to healing degenerative diseases, they fail. In fact, they are not too bright. They may have ten years of university schooling, but you can get brainwashed to a point where you do not look at the gray areas; they tend to go down the road until they run right off the cliff.

Many people die from IVs if they are infused too quickly. If you have fourteen pints of blood, you cannot put eighteen in there; it has to come out, otherwise you will suffer complications such as heart failure or pneumonia induced by the IV fluid.

Electrolyte imbalances take place also, then you will hear them come out and say, "Mrs. Jones expired from heart failure." Well, they might have caused it.

In my mother's case, when she had cirrhosis of the liver, they told me I could not turn it around. I did turn it around, because I have the CAT scan that shows new liver tissue regenerating. I relieved jaundice in less than two weeks, and in two years she was perfect, an eighty-five-year-old woman. She developed a bladder infection; at that time I was not in this field, but I was pretty knowledgeable. She told me she was getting chills and I noticed that she had a one-hundred-two-degree fever, so I brought her to the hospital and they discovered she had a bladder infection. They killed my mother with an IV.

They ran glucose into her, and it was supposed to have been infused over eleven hours. It was put in, in an hour and a half and she went into a sugar coma and she died. That is only one case. A few years back, the doctors went on strike in California. They were on strike for thirty days and the death rate went down. Then, when they went back, the death rate leveled off to what it normally is. Does that tell you something?

JIMMY: Yeah.

DR. RUCCIO: There were many unnecessary surgeries performed on women, like hysterectomies, and they get away with that. The medical profession has a way of covering its tracks. When the medical profession says medical records are private, that's because they protect their own interest by not having that information out. They kind of bury that sort of thing. Do you have any questions you want to ask me?

JIMMY: Dr. Lane talks in his first book about how there is no hard evidence comparing the effectiveness of the shark cartilage with or without conventional therapies. I'm a perfect example.

DR. RUCCIO: His new piece that he has done, he mentions what chemotherapy does. Of course, one can't tell you not to use chemotherapy, but they can give you an opinion like I did. I can't legally tell anyone, "Look, I don't want you to use chemotherapy." That's their choice. Shark cartilage works very well on cases that are one and two, and there are also some stage-four cases on prostate cancer that do well.

Stage four on some breast cancer, and then there are some aggressive breast cancers. Nothing works all the time, even shark cartilage may not work for everyone. But what we're finding is that it is working for quite a lot of people. There are a lot of doctors out there that are gathering the information. Medical documents, which I would consider scientific, as long as it's a medical doctor and it's not played around with and altered. It's out there, and that's what Dr. Lane is gathering.

JIMMY: Does he now have more evidence of shark cartilage working without the conventional therapies?

DR. RUCCIO: Oh yeah, this is what's happening. Most of the people, with the exception of a few, will do chemotherapy and radiation. We usually get them when they're a basket case. They have already had surgery, chemotherapy, and the radiation failed. So it's a little harder. For instance, I have a guy who has lung cancer up in New York State and his tumors are gone.

A few weeks ago, he had some bleeding; he's coughing up blood he thought was a tumor. I suggested that maybe he go back to his physician, because I thought it could be pleurisy or pneumonia. Upon examination, it was pleurisy, and he's still responding pretty well. He's not taking chemotherapy, because they told him they couldn't do any more. In fact, they wanted to send a hospice to his home. That tells you right there, they threw the towel in on him.

JIMMY: What's a hospice?

DR. RUCCIO: Usually, when you are on your way out, they'll come in and they usually deal with pain management. There are some cases that I found where people were given morphine when they didn't even need it. Morphine causes complications like constipation, loss of appetite, and nausea. If a patient can't eat, he is eventually going to die from starvation. That goes on also. Maybe their intentions are well meant. To start somebody on morphine when they're not even in pain, I question that. I have my own reasons why I think they do that. I just don't think it's right.

I had people on morphine who followed an alternative protocol and they're off morphine. They had to be weaned, but they're off it. Of course, there are some that you just can't get off.

JIMMY: How many people are out there like me, that absolutely will not go the conventional route and just go with the shark cartilage? This is the proof in the pudding right there.

DR. RUCCIO: In the cases that I have dealt with, I would say twenty percent. The other eighty percent had chemotherapy or radiation which failed, and now they're trying other remedies.

JIMMY: So you think the people that didn't take the radiation and just went strictly with the shark cartilage in the beginning did better or improved faster.

DR. RUCCIO: Well, I could only say that the cases that I have documented here, backed up by MRIs and CAT Scans, I would say maybe they're better off. I cannot legally tell a person—I have to make this clear to you, Jimmy—I cannot tell a person not to use chemotherapy or radiation, which I don't do. I tell them what I think can happen. I tell them that before they do their chemotherapy, they should get the pharmaceutical inserts and see what all the downsides are. The doctors will usually give you a computer paper which will indicate some of the side effects, but they don't tell you them all. The pharmaceutical insert will tell you everything. Then, I tell them to base their decision on the best information.

Whether they use chemotherapy or not, I will still help them out to try to keep their body nutritionally strong. That's the whole key. If you're weak, you have no fight left. You have to keep the body strong and keep the red blood and white blood–cell count up. You have to make sure their chemistry is right.

Some of these doctors are really good, but they don't check the chemistry. Sometimes they don't turn over every stone. I don't know whether it's because there are too many people for them to handle, or it's a money thing. When Jimmy Blanco's gone, there is another Jimmy Blanco to fill his place. This is the whole thing in a nutshell. If you're an oncologist for twenty or thirty years, you know what works and what doesn't work.

JIMMY: I believe only a fool would try the same thing over and over and expect a different response. If you know chemotherapy doesn't work for brain tumors, why would anyone keep suggesting it? Do they expect a different response, or are they milking the insurance companies?

DR. RUCCIO: In lung cancer, usually eighty-five to eighty-eight percent of the people don't make it, so why are you using chemotherapy? Because it doesn't work. They'll probably live longer if you leave them alone, but they're not going to let the money go down the tubes. They're going to grab all the bucks they can. That's what it's all about.

Now they're losing people to alternatives, so they're trying to become nutritionists overnight. They don't have the degree on the wall, they have about an hour of nutrition, and yet they're going to set my standards? They're going to tell me what to do? When I'm trained in the field? That's wrong, but that's what they're doing. That's where the law has to be changed.

There are many, many health professionals out there. Some are physicians, some are non-physicians, and some non-physicians are better than the doctors, as far as maintaining a person's nutritional status.

JIMMY: Last time we spoke, you said that the medical field calls your field quackery.

DR. RUCCIO: They are the biggest quacks around. I'm going to tell you what proves that — if they were not quacks, why are they now teaching this in some medical schools? Actually, what they're doing now is jumping on the bandwagon. Medical doctors are politicians; they put their finger in the air and whichever way the wind is blowing, they want to be on the right side of the issue.

Columbia University and the University of Arizona are now teaching, and a few more in the Midwest. There are at least eight to ten that are teaching new medical doctors this. I'm happy; what that does is it enhances my degree. Naturopathic oncologists at one time were not accredited, but they are accredited now. Even if they are not accredited, they were still pioneering in this field where the medical estab-lishment was out there calling everyone names.

I would like to see a class-action suit and an antitrust suit filed against the medical profession, like the chiropractors did. The medical profession has the pharmaceutical companies behind them and they have the support of the politicians, whom they go down and lobby and put money into their campaigns. These politicians don't care because they don't understand; they're not doctors themselves.

I know a few politicians that got sick in Washington and they're doing alternatives. It's amazing, isn't it? Yet, they will not change the law throughout the land. If you're a medical doctor, you do your medical stuff, that's your turf. If a person is an alternative doctor, he has a right to do his thing.

JIMMY: You mentioned before that, in your opinion, the chemotherapy kills the patients before the cancer does.

DR. RUCCIO: In some cases, not in all cases. I definitely know chemotherapy weakens them. A perfect example is depression of bone marrow. So now they get on television looking for bone marrow donors for the individual. That shows you that the chemotherapy has dire, dire dangerous complications which may kill you before the cancer does. What happens is the chemotherapy—not all chemotherapy does this—you're either vomiting, they're nauseous, they can't eat. If you can't eat, you're going to die. You're either going to die from the cancer, the treatment, or from not being able to eat. There's no way you can fight off disease if you can't keep yourself nutritionally sound or strong. I think you'll agree with that. You know what this is about? Jimmy, this is basic common sense. That's all it is. Some people are blind by the almighty dollar and they push common sense in the corner.

JIMMY: In your own opinion, is it better to bypass radiation and chemotherapy and just go with shark cartilage?

DR. RUCCIO: That's my opinion.

JIMMY: In your opinion; I know you can't recommend it.

DR. RUCCIO: Yes, but don't bypass surgery, though. Radiation temporarily shrinks the tumor because it does kill some cells, but it also dehydrates that tumor. It's almost like a microwave. You put a piece of meat in it that weighs one pound and it comes out a half a pound. That's a temporary fix.

As far as chemotherapy, you're going to kill off good cells and the bad cells, too, or the chemotherapy is going to cause heart failure, kidney failure, and organ damage. That doesn't make any sense to me at all. I think what's going on in this country is that people are being led to the slaughterhouse. You have to kind of feel sorry for them, because they're frightened and they're terrorized and scared. They don't know what to do, because we were all trained and all raised to be traditional. I was until I started opening my eyes and saying, "What are these guys doing?"

I praise them and compliment them when it comes to a life-threatening situation. I think the surgeons in this country are the best in the world. I think they're good guys. I get a lot of cooperation from the surgeons. I don't get too much cooperation with the oncologists. In fact, one woman asked her oncologist to call me and he had to refuse. Well, if he thinks he knows more than me about this, he's got a long way to go.

General practitioners are pretty good, but of course, some of them are scared to death. They're afraid of the FDA. As long as the FDA approves something, even if it kills you, they're going to do it. That's what's wrong. I am a pioneer in this field. I don't want to be above the doctors, I want to be able to walk into a hospital and be able to assist them. Also, make some recommendations and things like that. It's not going to come in my lifetime, but it may eventually come. When they see that naturopathic consultants are not a threat, that's when they're going to open the door. I just have to believe that it's a money thing. You can't make money if people are well.

Good nutritionists could keep people out of the hospital, but hospitals don't want that. They only make money by selling their beds. By the way, they're having trouble filling their beds. That's why many hospitals are merging today. These HMO doctors are getting residuals not to send you to a specialist. I have a lady in New York who's having trouble getting treated because of the HMOs.

That's crazy, she's paying her premiums. I ask her why she can't go to her hospital to have this or that check; she says they won't pay for it. I tell her that she ought to call the prosecutor's office and file a complaint. She should write some letters to Washington, DC, to the attorney general's office about what's going on, and hopefully she does that.

I live in a rental; I don't have a lot of money. I drive a 1990 car. Since 1992 I think I've consulted with about two thousand people, I have their names. If anyone was to call these people, not one person did I take a dime from. People ask, why do you do this? I'm interested in the research and I'm interested in proving the medical profession wrong. Because they killed my mother, and because I could get cancer, and so could those politicians and so could those doctors. I don't want to be in a situation where someone tells me that I have to take chemotherapy if I don't want it. Do you think a medical doctor has the right to tell you to go home and die when he thinks you're going to die?

JIMMY: No.

DR. RUCCIO: If the doctors tell you, "I think you ought to go out and live your life, go out and have a lot of fun because you have so much time to live," he's not God; he can't tell you how much time one has to live. Don't you think you should have the right to go seek out any other health professional that you want to talk to? A physician or non-physician?

JIMMY: Definitely. I am going to try my best to change that. I will try to get reimbursed for my alternative treatment. It is to the insurance company's benefit to cover a treatment that costs a fraction of what chemotherapy and radiation cost. Also, unlike conventional treatment, it works.

DR. RUCCIO: Okay. That's the point. There are many people told to go home and die, and they're wrong. The first case we had was from a major cancer center in New York. A seventy-two-year-old gentleman with esophageal cancer. They said he had three months to live. He was the first case that I worked with a medical doctor. I was teaching him alternatives in Bloomfield, New Jersey. Within six weeks we had calcification of a tumor that metastasized on his back. That case was on the *60 Minutes* program. There was a doctor who was on *60 Minutes* who wrote a book who's out there like he's a guru. When we went down there to show him this, he indicated that this was a delayed action from radiation a year and a half ago. Radiation doesn't last that long. That was the first case and no one has been consulting about shark cartilage longer than I have in the US.

I started in June of 1992. At that time, Dr. Lane had to go to Cuba for his research because no one would touch it here. This is when I started, and no one has more experience than me.

I don't care if they're doctors, geniuses, or rocket scientists, no one has worked with this as long as I have. My field should be recognized for its contributions. We shouldn't be on the outside looking in. Insurance companies have a chance of saving millions of dollars. Yet, if I consulted you, I would be considered a provider to the insurance companies.

Why not? If I saved them money, I should be recognized. In your particular case, how much money do you think the insurance companies save?

JIMMY: A lot! My limit is a million dollars. I could have very easily reached my limit if I chose to do so.

DR. RUCCIO: You should call them and ask them, "How much would it cost you if you were to be treating me for another year?"

JIMMY: So let me ask you. Why BeneFin?

DR. RUCCIO: Because I think it's the best product. All the sharks in the ocean are the same; what makes the BeneFin work is the processing. Some of these cartilages are cleaned with chemicals that make them carcinogenic in their own right. Others are not cleaning them well enough. There are some companies that you can actually see the blood in the capsule. Those are the kind of people that discredit my field. They're out for the buck. There is nothing wrong with making money, as long as you do the job.

Also, there are some companies that put sugar in. Now, suppose you're giving that cartilage to someone who's diabetic. There is a major company that puts sugar in shark cartilage, and they put down one hundred percent shark cartilage. It's not one hundred percent, it has sugar. There is liquid shark cartilage, which I have the chemical test here; Dr. Lane had it done. This company is claiming pure shark cartilage. Well, it's one percent shark cartilage and ninety-nine percent water. So this is what's going on out there. Everyone is jumping on Dr. Lane's coattails.

JIMMY: What about all this other cartilage I hear so much about, the bovine and the calf?

DR. RUCCIO: Dr. Lane and Dr. Prudden used to work together, and in my opinion, Dr. Prudden just picked the wrong horse. Bovine has some effect, but it's nowhere and no way near as strong as shark cartilage. Cows get cancer, and sharks, maybe one in a million get it. Draw your own conclusions as to what's the better product. I think the bovine might help on certain cancers, but it's not stronger than shark cartilage.

JIMMY: What are the other diseases shark cartilage is good for other than cancer?

DR. RUCCIO: It's good for arthritis.

JIMMY: Would you say it's good for any tumorous cancers?

DR. RUCCIO: Any? We know it's worked on adenocarcinomas, on certain breast cancers—some forms of breast cancers are more aggressive. We know it's worked on liver cancers, we know it works on brain tumors, but then there is a point of no return with brain tumors too. It depends on where the tumor is. All of this has to be taken into account.

I get calls from England, the Philippines, Bahamas, Canada, Chile, China. Right now, there must be at least eight hundred thousand to two million people using shark cartilage throughout the world. I think there are maybe two to three hundred thousand in the United States.

JIMMY: Can you tell me about the basic theory of anti-angiogenesis that makes shark cartilage work?

DR. RUCCIO: The hypothesis is that it's anti-angiogenic and the blood vessels atrophy and deprive the tumor of a blood supply. Now, we know we're right. There's a major hospital in New York that tried to make it injectable. If we were wrong, why has the anti-angiogenic theory become so popular now? Why is everyone looking at that?

Doctors aren't stupid; they see many patients that have failed chemotherapy and radiation. All of a sudden, they're taking cartilage and some other things, and to their surprise, they are getting better. They know what is going on, they know this has promise. It works in many cases; of course, there are some cases it doesn't work in. I have a case of a young man with testicular cancer that metastasized to the abdominal cavity and he had a tumor the size of a grapefruit. The mother called me to tell me her son was on his deathbed. He's now playing video games, going out to dinner, and the tumor has shrunk one inch. He had chemotherapy two years ago, and while he was on the chemotherapy, the tumor was growing. You have to take each case separately.

You can't bunch everyone up and say, oh, this is going to work on you. When I talk to them, I tell them right out—it may work, and it may not. This is an experimental thing. You have to use your own judgment. NO ONE HAS THE RIGHT TO TELL YOU TO GO HOME AND DIE! No one has that right. If someone tells you you're going to die, you must do whatever you have to do to try to save your life. I know that I've already saved people's lives, and you're one of them. When I look in the mirror every morning, I feel good about myself. My satisfaction comes from people like you, who call me and tell me, guess what, things are going well. I feel good about myself. My motive is not money. If my motive was money, I would own a new home and car. I would have everything else that a doctor has.

JIMMY: I don't know how religious you are, but I feel that God has guided me to you.

DR. RUCCIO: Look, I'm religious too. I believe God has put me here to do certain things. I had a pretty tough time in my life. My only satisfaction is to make my mark and to do some good for humanity. That makes me feel good. Some people feel good when they eat bubblegum. I feel good when people tell me that they got better from these terrible diseases out there. We don't know all the causes, but I believe it's environmental, and some may be genetic. Some may be chemically induced; for instance, drugs like estrogen can cause cancer, those kinds of things.

There are some antibiotics that depress the immune system and set you up to develop cancer. I believe a man should be able to live to be one hundred years old. You have the centurions that are out there now; if they could do it, then I would say the average American can do it.

People are living longer; they say it's because of medicine. I think it is the way you live. If you listen to these old folks, they'll tell you what they're eating. They're either not smoking or they're not in the type of environment that causes problems. They are usually calm types of people.

JIMMY: With no stress.

DR. RUCCIO: With no stress. They are kind of religious and they live a good, clean life. I believe this all plays a part in us living longer.

DR. RUCCIO: I believe that I've been, maybe, chosen to tell this story. Maybe God chose me because He knows my personality. He knows that I am strong-minded and when I put my mind to something, it gets done. I also believe He has given me the strength that I needed. I've experienced many miracles up until now.

DR. RUCCIO: You're a pretty lucky guy; something is happening here. Getting back to the medical profession, no one wants to take away anything from them. If a person needs surgery, any health professional should advise them to do so. The location of the tumors means a lot. It could be on a major blood vessel. When taking shark cartilage, in some cases the tumor will swell, because if you deprive the tumor of a blood supply, it's the same as if you were to put a tourniquet on the tip of your finger. Eventually, your finger will begin to swell and throb. If you go and have a CAT scan while that's happening, and that usually happens between eight to twelve weeks, if you go in to see the doctor, he'll tell you the tumor is growing. It may be growing in some cases, but what I'm finding is that tumors swell. Usually, by the fourth or fifth month, you go in for another CAT scan and the results will show no change. No change is a plus; it means it's not growing anymore.

Since I've been doing this, the best thing to come along for cancer has been shark cartilage. Nothing beats shark cartilage. When people use chemotherapy and radiation, they become nutritionally compromised or damaged and you have to try to build them up and get them going again. If you have someone that's been vomiting for two months with diarrhea, they're weak. They're dehydrated and a whole lot of things could happen.

You have to worry if you're going to die of malnutrition, dehydration, organ damage, heart failure, or kidney failure caused by various types of chemotherapy. Blood clots in their legs, then they put a screen in—a filter—I mean this is stupid! This is totally, really stupid! I have cancer, I have enough problems, and then I'm going in to do chemotherapy wanting to be helped and the chemotherapy causes a million other problems. It is really stupid.

I don't mind if a person does chemotherapy and radiation; I'll take them on. Usually, I get them when they're done with it. They ask me what could be done, and I tell them. I definitely indicate they have to be monitored by a medical doctor for CAT scans, MRIs, and whatever is necessary to follow the case. That's the intelligent and responsible way to do this, and I consider myself a pretty responsible guy. Some doctors don't want to follow the case because they're doing this or that. Why won't they follow it? My only reasoning is that they don't want this to work, and they don't want it medically documented.

If they do, it becomes a scientific document. I urge your readers to question their doctors about all these types of things. If they are doing an alternative, they should demand that it is documented on the radiological report, which would then become a scientific document.

So, Jimmy, if any of your readers are interested in my protocol, or any doctors with an open mind want to contact me, I would be glad to help out in any way that I could.[†]

[†] Dr. Dante Ruccio passed away in 2009.

⚜ 15 ⚜

Email to Dr. Chandak

I began to challenge this theory over the internet. I emailed Dr. Puneet Chandak, the President and Medical Director at Silicon Valley Medical Imaging in San Jose, California. I wrote:

> I think all the so-called experts have missed the boat when it comes to treating glioblastoma multiforme. I know of a person who has a grade IV and has brushed aside the doctors and treated himself. Ten months later, he has no recurrence. Do you think that is possible? Well, believe it.

His response:

Dear Jimmy Blanco,

I agree. Yes, "miracles," such as what you have described, though uncommon, are not nonexistent. These occurrences generate significant interest and produce many thought-provoking questions regarding the current understanding or practice of modern medicine; however, they do not occur as often, and cannot usually be repeated under a controlled clinical setting. As a result, our current understanding of such highly unusual and unexpected outcomes or occurrences is highly insufficient, and we will need more time to probe them enough and understand them in a more scientific way, before being able to utilize them routinely in our practices. As physicians, our objective is to understand, prevent, and cure disease, and to reduce or eliminate pain and suffering. Physicians today do not disregard such incidents as freak occurrences only. In fact, several physicians today encourage and/or advocate alternative treatments that can help cure disease or improve the quality of their patients' lives. Almost all remedies were initially unknown to us and came from understanding how some plant, or experimental drug, or procedure, or behavior, etc. changes the outcome of a disease. It has been a long process and emerged over a period of several hundred years. Personally, I wish I had the time, opportunity, or the means to study all such phenomena.

Good wishes,
Puneet Chandak, MD

I was very surprised that this doctor went into so much detail in explaining to me why modern medicine has not progressed in the fight against terminal illness.

In his closing thoughts he said, "Personally, I wish I had the time, opportunity, or the means to study all such phenomena." This doctor sounds like a person who really cares, and I know there are many more like him. He wishes he had the *time, opportunity,* and *means* to study all such phenomena.

My question is *why* don't doctors who care about finding answers have more resources to pursue loose ends and medical miracles? Why don't we have some of our tax dollars go to a research team staffed by inquisitive doctors like this one? Have them turn every stone and find out why some people are surviving while others are not. I think it will be money well spent. It's a lot cheaper than continuing to flip the bill for all the radiation and chemotherapy treatments.‡

---

‡ When Jamie contacted Dr. Chandak for the purposes of this book, more than twenty-five years after this email was sent, Dr. Chandak expressed amazement that Jimmy lived eight years after his diagnosis and said he remembered corresponding with him. Dr. Chandak expressed thanks to Jamie for finishing this book, saying it could give people hope that stories like Jimmy's are possible.

✤16✤

Dos and Don'ts for a New Cancer Patient

First, I'd like to say that I am not a doctor, nutritionist, or dietitian. I hold no degree in alternative therapies. The only therapy I am licensed in is respiratory therapy, which I have worked in for the last thirteen years.

I don't pass myself off as an authority in anything. I am just a cancer patient who is self-motivated. I am in a persistent search to find answers to questions I need to survive my so-called incurable disease.

So here are some of my dos and don'ts for the newly diagnosed cancer patient. You might say, "I'm not a cancer patient." Well, I wasn't either before October 26, 1995.

I purchased a new van one month before I was diagnosed and they asked me if I wanted disability insurance that would pay off the car in the event I was disabled. I looked at my wife and said, "Disabled? I'm thirty-six years old and have never been sick in my life. No way," and I didn't buy it. It was only a dollar, but I thought nothing could ever happen to me. Only other people become disabled.

No one knows what's going to happen tomorrow. I was walking around with a seven-centimeter tumor in my brain and I didn't even know it. You might have a friend or family member that is newly diagnosed. This may be helpful to them. When I was a boy in the scouts, our motto was "Be Prepared."

Please use your own judgment as to whether these are helpful.

DOs	DON'Ts
• Do get a second, third, and fourth opinion on your diagnosis and prognosis.	• Don't listen to your doctor's first prognosis; they could be wrong.
• Keep a positive and open mind. If you have to, go to a hypnotist to help you relax and get you into a positive state of mind. You can also listen to meditation tapes, which I found very helpful.	• Avoid putting yourself in a negative state of mind.
• Research every possible alternative for your type of cancer.	• Don't let them pressure or scare you into rushing. Some treatments respond better without radiation and chemotherapy, so do your research first.
• Utilize visualization. See yourself destroying the tumor. I often pictured myself inside my brain blasting my tumor with a ray gun.	• Don't blame anyone for your cancer or tumor. Don't ask God, "Why me?"
• Believe that everything happens for a reason and is for the best.	• If you think you're becoming depressed, seek treatment for yourself and your family. Don't let negativity beat you.
• Pray a lot and go to your church, synagogue, or mosque. Wherever you feel comfortable worshiping.	• Don't alienate your friends and family, because they love you and are suffering just as much as you are.
• Believe and ask God to	• Don't be so proud that you

heal you. If anyone can do it, it's Him. Remember, your mind is very powerful. You must believe that you are going to beat the odds.	won't allow anyone to help you financially or otherwise. You may be hurting someone's feelings.
• Try to focus on others' needs before your own. It is good for the soul and will take your mind off your problems. No matter how sick you are, there is always someone worse off.	• Don't aggravate yourself with the problems of daily living. Let someone else take charge if you can.
• Try to get away for a while if you can.	• Don't refuse to go to any house of worship you are invited to. If people are praying for you to recover, it's only common decency to say thank you. It doesn't matter what religion they are.
• Inform yourself about side effects, and try to avoid medications and treatments with adverse effects when possible.	• Don't let the doctor be the sole maker of your medical decisions. Be an active participant in your health plan. Find a doctor who understands this and is willing to have discussions with you.
• Learn as much as you can from other cancer survivors. They can offer more wisdom than the doctors can. Also, become a good listener.	• Don't feel pressured to do anything you don't feel comfortable with. It's your body and your life.

• Contact as many alternative doctors and clinics as possible. Get opinions from all of them, then decide what route you should take.	• Don't sit at home and rot. The more active you are, the better chance you have of recovering.
• Listen to your gut feeling when it comes to choosing a treatment plan.	• Don't be embarrassed, ashamed, or hesitant in telling your doctor exactly what you want and don't want. If he feels uncomfortable with what you want to do, find another doctor.
• Thank God every morning that you wake up. Pray that He will guide you in the right direction and give you strength to overcome your ordeal. Trust that He will.	• Avoid things that will aggravate you.
• Go to the beach and walk along the edge of the water. Think about beautiful things that make you happy.	• Don't feel sorry for yourself. This is an unproductive behavior.
• Have a massage therapist come to your house. I did this three times a week and found it very helpful.	• Don't force things to happen. You may be setting yourself up for a big disappointment. If a treatment doesn't work, find another one that will.

If I tell you that I'm completely recovered, I'd be lying to you. I am still recovering from a very serious and traumatic surgery.

I still have cerebral spinal fluid and blood accumulated in my right frontal lobe. This makes me very dizzy and weak. I have headaches, memory loss, and twitches. I have good days and bad days.

The fact that I am still alive, as of this writing, one year and six months later, is a major accomplishment. Especially when the doctors only gave me three months to live and no hope of ever being cured with or without radiation and chemotherapy. These are all good signs that I may have a chance to beat this thing.

The more time I spend with my kids, the more I feel that God has put children on this Earth so we can learn what our relationship with Him is like.

God loves us the same way we love our own children. He wants the best for us. He forgives us in a similar way we do our children. He makes us look at things from his point of view when we teach and discipline our children. We are all His children and are taught, disciplined, forgiven, and most of all, loved by Him.

Life is a learning process from start to finish. Each phase of life prepares us for the next until we go back to our Father in Heaven. We all have our time to go home. Trust in God's will.

❧ 17 ❧

MRI Helpful Hints

F or those individuals who have never had to do an MRI (magnetic resonance imaging), consider yourself lucky. I hope you never have to perform this terrible procedure, especially if you are claustrophobic like me. It feels like being buried alive. The patient is placed in a tube that he or she barely fits in. He or she must remain motionless for almost an hour, staring straight at the top of the tube that is just inches from your face. Some people don't have a problem with that, but I wasn't one of them. I would scream for them to pull me out within seconds of being rolled in. If you are one of those chickens like me, I have some helpful hints. This seemed to work for me, the ultimate claustrophobic, and if it worked for me, it will work for anyone.

- Shop around for the most modern facility with up-to-date equipment. There are now open MRI facilities, which is great, but it is not always possible to get into one of these.
- Speak with the person in charge of the department and ask for a tour.
- Compare the sizes of the machines. Some are bigger than others. A few inches can make a big difference.
- Make sure they have a mirror that is positioned correctly so you can see out.

- Make sure they have the tools to protect your ears. It's very loud.
- Some facilities have music you can listen to. This is very helpful, but the noise is usually louder.
- The best facilities will have a video screen where you can watch a movie through the mirror.
- It's a good idea to bring your own meditation or nature sounds tape.
- Another great idea is to keep your eyes closed the entire time. Picture yourself somewhere else like the beach or wherever you like best.
- This is an excellent time to use visualization. Picture yourself miniaturized and destroying whatever ailment you have. Concentrate on healing.
- It's also a great time to do some praying. Ask God to help guide you through these hard times. Ask God to heal you and everyone else who may be sick.
- Remove all negative thoughts from your mind.
- What I found most helpful was to take a melatonin a half hour before the procedure, almost guaranteeing you will sleep through the entire procedure. The day of your MRI, try to be awake early, long before the procedure, so you are more tired.

Everyone is different, so use the method that works best for you.

After the procedure, always ask for a copy of your MRI for your personal records. Most modern facilities will be able to give them to you on the spot. If not, go to medical records a few days later, and they must give them to you at no charge. I hope these tips will be useful and will make this uncomfortable procedure more palatable.

⚜18⚜

Wake Up, America

I was going to prove to the medical establishment that there is a way to beat cancer. Where there is a will, there is always a way.

This was my mission, to survive and surprise the doctors. Force them to look at alternatives as a way to save lives. They need to open their eyes to what works and stop wasting taxpayer money trying to perfect radiation and chemotherapy. They've spent our money for over fifty years and millions of Americans are still dying. America needs to wake up and demand answers from its elected officials. We've spent billions on weapons of mass destruction, trillions on star war defense systems that do not work. What kind of commitment have we made to find a cure for cancer?

Isn't our tax money better spent on helping people instead of finding better ways of killing them?

We made a commitment to go to the moon and accomplished it in less than a decade. Let's make a commitment to change our medical system so that it is more oriented toward helping the sick instead of what it is today, nothing but a business. Whenever one talks about changes in the medical system, immediately they are branded a communist or a left-wing liberal. Let's put aside the name-calling and politics.

Republicans and Democrats alike are afflicted with cancer and other debilitating diseases. The fact is that we are probably the only nation in the world that doesn't have nationalized medicine.

Canada, Great Britain, France, Germany—I could go on and on. These countries are not communist.

I would like to see real progress in improving healthcare as we know it. There has been a lot of talk of belt-tightening and achieving more at less cost. I would like to see that I have made a difference and my suffering amounted to some good in this area. I can see an America where doctors focus more on the prevention of disease instead of waiting until the damage is done, after which it may be too late to do anything.

Prevention will significantly lower healthcare costs. I could see how this would not only cut healthcare costs, but insurance premiums as well. I may be asking for too much if I say I would like to see physicians care more about their patients than money. I would like to see an America where naturopathic doctor consultants like Dr. Dante Ruccio will have the opportunity to work peacefully and in conjunction with the mainstream medical physician.

I would like to see an America where the consumer is allowed the opportunity to choose the type of treatment he or she feels will be beneficial to themselves. If conventional medicine had all the answers, people would not be searching for alternatives. Why can't they just admit that they don't know everything and there just might be something to these alternatives that are helping so many people? Why must they be at each other's throats?

According to a National Institutes of Health publication called *Alternative Medicine: Expanding Medical Horizons*, in a January 1995 report on Alternative Medical Systems and Practices in the United States, "Many alternative practitioners face numerous economic, political, and scientific barriers that block their acceptance by mainstream biomedicine."[17] On the

---

[17] National Institutes of Health (US), Workshop on Alternative Medicine, "Alternative Medicine: Expanding Medical Horizons. A Report to the National Institutes of Health on Alternative Medical Systems and Practices in the United States," 1992.

other hand, some alternative medical practitioners do not expect to be brought into the fold. Rather, they just want the opportunity to work alongside mainstream medical practitioners and to be allowed to offer consumers alternative healthcare options.

Consumers, however, are not waiting for mainstream science to give them a "green light" on many alternative treatments before using them.

Surveys have demonstrated that most people who opt to use alternative treatments believe that conventional medicine has not adequately addressed their needs. People like me, or those with chronic, debilitating illnesses like arthritis, epilepsy, chronic pain, cancer, and AIDS. People often are attracted to alternative medicine practitioners who emphasize the patient's role in the healing process. In contrast, most conventional medical practitioners take the patient out of the loop. They want to dictate to the patient what they have to do. They practically make the decision for the patient by not being educated in other possible alternative treatments that may be better suited for the patient's recovery.

According to the same NIH report, studies also show that individuals who seek out and use alternative medical treatment tend to be better educated and more affluent. Researchers write, "Thus, the stereotype of the alternative medicine consumer as an uneducated, poor person succumbing to the sideshow lures of quacks and charlatans appears to be greatly overblown."[18]

The report finds, "One of the simplest and most effective ways to significantly lower health care costs and thus increase access is through a major focus on preventive medicine. . . . In this clinical arena, many of the alternative health care systems

---

https://chiro.org/alt_med_abstracts/FULL/Expanding_Medical_Horizons_UPDATE/index.shtml.

[18] Ibid.

may have much to offer. Homeopathic and naturopathic physicians, for example, strongly advise their patients about diet and other health-promoting lifestyle choices as a matter of routine care. In contrast, many conventional physicians do not routinely give such advice until a patient has already become chronically ill, by which time the patient may need expensive high-tech surgery and face a lifetime of expensive drug therapy."[19]

Another major factor contributing to the sky-rocketing healthcare cost in this country is the amount of time involved in officially certifying a drug or medical intervention as clinically effective and safe. It takes millions of dollars and sometimes many, many years before a potentially life-saving drug or intervention makes its way through the complex federal approval process. That same process too often ignores or discounts potentially valuable Canadian, European, and Asian data that could significantly shorten the assessment process.

The challenge for healthcare policymakers and federal regulators is to ensure the public's access to the most effective treatments available. Certainly, patients should have recourse if it can be shown that their practitioners or the treatment they offer has no clinical or psychological benefit. At the same time, patients with debilitating severe or chronic illnesses should have the right to have access to—as well as insurance to cover—an alternative therapy they believe offers them relief or a cure.

---

[19] Ibid.

Jamie's Epilogue

My father stopped writing this book around the time of his third surgery in the year 2000. By then, looking at computer screens became too difficult for him.

From the time of my father's first surgery in 1995, when he was given seventeen weeks to live, he did not have a recurrence of his tumor again until 1998, three years later. He had surgery to remove it and continued his regimen of shark cartilage and supplements. The tumors returned again in the year 2000, and because he refused a protocol of chemo wafers, surgeons in Miami refused to treat him and he was forced to go out of state for his surgery to Cedars-Sinai Medical Center in Los Angeles, California. The tumor returned again in 2002 when he had a final surgery at Kendall Regional Medical Center in Miami. By 2003, there were numerous tumors in his brain and around his body that were inoperable. He passed away on November 22, 2003, eight years to the day that he took his first dose of shark cartilage.

This timeline is extraordinary given that these tumors normally recur within two to three months without treatment and Jimmy Blanco never once participated in traditional protocols of chemotherapy or radiation nor did he participate in clinical trials or receive any mainstream medical interventions besides surgery for treatment of his GBMs.

There are four aspects to my father's self-care that I believe were extremely important to his longevity and beneficial to anyone fighting a major diagnosis: Spirituality, Mental Fortitude, Nutrition, and Shark Cartilage.

Let's begin with the last one.

Shark Cartilage

Shark cartilage is not the only supplement my father took but it is the one he credits most with slowing the growth of his tumors. Whether actual or placebo effect, it's difficult to know for sure. What I do know for sure is there's no way he should have lived as long as he did, and shark cartilage was at the heart of his self-treatment.

When I set out to write the epilogue for this book, I was discouraged by what I found. After refusing to remove the claim that shark cartilage can treat cancer from its labels, a US federal court in 2004 ordered Dr. William Lane's company to destroy all of its shark cartilage products and reimburse its customers.[20] Only some of the product was kept for clinical research.

I discovered that it was now very difficult to find high-quality powdered shark cartilage in the amount and purity similar to what my father had used to treat himself. My stomach sank thinking how difficult it would be for newly diagnosed patients to get ahold of what my father believed had worked for him.

I started reaching out to current naturopathic cancer doctors and those from my father's past to talk about his preferred self-treatment. Unfortunately, Dr. Dante Ruccio, who advised my father on how to take shark cartilage, passed away in 2009 from a cancer diagnosis of his own, after a long battle with the disease.

I tried interviewing Dr. William Lane, the author of *Sharks Don't Get Cancer*, back in 2008 when I was a student journalist at Emerson College for a public affairs piece I was putting together on natural medicine. What I found was a broken man. He said he

---

[20] United States v. Lane Labs - USA, Inc., 324 F. Supp. 2d 547 (D.N.J. 2004).

was glad that his product had helped my father, but he was not legally able to make any comments or claims about the health benefits, cancer or otherwise, of shark cartilage.

Dr. Lane passed away in 2011.

As I explained in the introduction to this book, the FDA became interested in shark cartilage back in the early '90s when Dr. Lane directed a seemingly successful human study in Cuba on twenty-nine advanced cancer patients who failed under all conventional treatments and were receiving shark cartilage.

His study was featured on CBS's *60 Minutes* with Mike Wallace in February and July of 1993. Once it became popularized, the snake oil salesmen pounced. My father shared in this book his own story of Dr. Lane saving him after being sold overpriced, phony, "injectable" shark cartilage.

In an interview with Healthy.net, Dr. Lane himself warned about scammers, saying: "The *60 Minutes* show did my research a lot of good, but it had a bad side as well. Bad because it suddenly brought in about thirty new competitors. Some of them are good products but some of them are not. It seems odd that something that took me years of research to develop took others less than two weeks. You can't even run tests in two weeks! Yet, there were thirty new products on the market in about two weeks. Half of these overnight products were half sugar. There seem to be more sharks on the land than there are in the ocean."[21]

Dr. Lane claimed to have seen a positive response, whether halting tumor growth or improving a sense of well-being, from nearly one hundred percent of patients with various types of cancer he treated in Cuba. His time in Cuba is the centerpiece of a documentary called *The Politics of Cancer*. But his methodology was criticized by the scientific community and his studies were never published in peer-reviewed journals. His study was not a

---

[21] Richard A. Passwater, PhD, "Shark Cartilage and Cancer, Revisited:A follow-up interview," Healthy.net, 1993. https://healthy.net/2019/08/26/shark-cartilage-and-cancer-revisiteda-follow-up-interview/.

controlled study and his assessment of patients amounted to self-reported interviews with the subjects.

When his results could not be reproduced by American medical trials, the FDA ordered Dr. Lane's shark cartilage company to remove the claims about treating cancer from its labels. Dr. Lane refused to remove the claims, pushing instead for more research to be done first, but ultimately the government shut down the production of all the company's products.

The problem is, as I've stated before, that the government took that extreme action despite inconclusive and incomplete American clinical trials, *none* of which were performed on newly diagnosed patients as the sole or main therapy without being administered alongside the chemo and radiation that proponents of shark cartilage contended destroyed the natural treatment's efficacy.

Dr. Michael Greger from NutritionFacts.org makes an excellent video outlining many of the main clinical trials involving shark cartilage, and you can find detailed information on all of those trials via the National Institutes of Health on ClinicalTrials.gov.

One of the doctors who treated my father and is still alive as of this writing is Dr. Eduardo A. Recio Roura of Spain. Between 2000 and 2003, Dr. Recio prescribed and mailed injectable therapies to my father, which my mother administered. I was able to have a brief conversation with Dr. Recio in Spanish on the phone.

Dr. Recio expressed that the '90s and early 2000s were an era in which shark cartilage was widely used, but that he never personally prescribed it. He believes that there have been advances that could possibly be more helpful in the fight against cancer since that time than shark cartilage.

You can read more of my insights on the latest exciting clinical trials and glioblastoma super-survivors in the introduction to this book.

Shark cartilage is still found in health food stores, mostly as a supplement used to help treat osteoarthritis, plaque psoriasis, diabetic damage to the retina, wound healing, and inflammation of the intestines.

I do not claim to be an expert; I do not have a medical degree and I am not a medical researcher. I can only testify to the true experience of my father and the eight incredible years he fought the deadliest brain cancer diagnosis without relying on traditional cancer protocols.

Whether the shark cartilage actually slowed the growth of the tumors or my father's strong belief in it, combined with the other natural medicines, herbs, nutrition changes, and his enduring spirituality contributed to his longer remissions, we may never know. But my father's steadfast faith, in general, was a great source of strength for him.

Spirituality

I believe faith was also one of the largest components of my father's healing. From the moment he declared before his congregation, a month after his diagnosis, that God was going to heal him without chemo or radiation, my father set his mind, body, and soul on the path to receive that miracle.

I remember when I was a kid how he would leave for a day to sit on the beach and have conversations with God. Or he'd take me back to Tropical Christian School, long after I stopped attending classes there, to spend a few hours in their chapel. I'd sit in a back pew and he'd sit in the front, and I would often cry my sincere prayers there about anything and everything.

He took us to many kinds of churches, some louder than others, but I don't think he was looking to believe anything that was thrown at him. He was seeking out a genuine truth for himself, for something that resonated. I remember we went to one of those churches where the pastor puts his hand on your head and yells a few words and people fall convulsing. The pastor put his hands on my father and pushed his head back, but my father didn't fall. The pastor tried pushing him again, harder this time, and shouting louder. When my father didn't fall again, the pastor left him standing and kept moving down the line. We didn't go back to that church, but we did return to many others. That's not a negative indictment of those kinds of churches, it just didn't resonate with my father.

He went to every church he was invited to, and tried many on his own, always open-minded and looking for truth that felt genuine to him. The Catholic church near our home was one of his favorites. There he used to get bottles of holy water to drink. He put faith in that water and prayed for healing whenever he drank it. I've never heard of anyone doing that, but he did. He sought out his own journey of faith. He put himself in God's hands and believed.

But it wasn't easy. Every setback was devastating. Every time the tumors returned, or after brain surgery when he was a little less himself, the sickness took its toll on him and our family over a long period of time. Life is messy and hard. But he never lost faith, because he could see that every day that he was alive was a miracle. It doesn't look like a made-for-TV movie. It's what you choose to do with that pain that matters. God's Son and His servants in the Bible were often those who suffered the most to bring a message of hope to the people. There is virtue in suffering gracefully.

Speaking of the beauty of suffering, among the bigger spiritual influences on my father was the story of his favorite saint, St. Francis of Assisi, founder of the Franciscan Order. I recommend everyone read his story.

He was born in 1182 and baptized by his mother as Giovanni after John the Baptist. His father, who had been away on business, returned and was enraged because he did not want his son to be a Godly man, he wanted him to be a businessman and share his love of France, so his father renamed him Francesco.

Francis enjoyed a very rich and easy life and admitted that he lived in sin as a young man. He was always affable and extremely well-liked. He sought wealth and the glory of battle. When Assisi declared battle on a neighboring city, he took up the mantle of knighthood. When all the forces of Assisi were slaughtered, he was captured and ransomed for his money.

Not the most upstanding guy yet, huh? But I believe that God's forgiveness is greater than our sins.

After being a prisoner, he knew that he wanted more from life but didn't know what. He gave himself again to partying.

Then, again in search of glory, he set off to fight as a knight in the Fourth Crusades, commissioning expensive armor and promising to return this time as a prince! But just one day into his journey he had a dream where God told him he was doing the wrong thing and to return home, redirecting his misplaced heroism. Francis did return home, where he was shamed, ridiculed, and called a coward by those who had loved and admired him all his life. Had they truly ever loved him, or just the money in his pocket? But he found joy unlike any he had experienced in following God's word, a total liberation.

His transformation didn't happen overnight.

A twenty-five-year-old Francis spent more and more time in prayer and went to a cave, where he wept for his sins. He felt God's peace and joy, but he still had a business to run and other responsibilities to his family. It was during this time, while out riding in the countryside, that Francis came face to face with a leper.

He was repulsed by the leper's appearance and smell, but regardless, he jumped down and kissed his hand. When his gesture of peace was returned, Francis was filled with joy. As he rode away, he turned around to wave goodbye and saw the leper had disappeared. Francis always considered it a test from God that he had passed.

Francis was praying at an ancient church in San Damiano when the story goes that he heard Christ on the crucifix speak to him. He heard Christ say, "Francis, repair my church."

He took it to mean the literal church crumbling around him, so Francis impulsively took fabric from his father's business, sold them, and gave the money to the church. His father, enraged, considered it a theft. Combined with his perceived cowardice, and disinterest in money, Francis's father dragged his son before the church's bishop, demanding the return of the money and for Francis to give up his claim as heir.

The bishop told Francis to give back the money because God would provide. Not only did he return the cash but he removed all his rich clothes, renounced his father, and embraced his Father in Heaven.

Wearing rags and living in the freezing woods, Francis began begging for stones to repair the church. He slept in the open, ate garbage, and loved God. He was always joyful and singing. When someone beat him and robbed him and left him in a ditch, he crawled back out and kept on singing. There was corruption in the church at the time and Francis began preaching a simpler, purer take on the Bible.

Soon Francis gained followers, and one day they gathered together to look in the Bible for direction. They prayed that His will would be revealed to them when they opened it. As Francis opened the Bible the first time, he read: *If you wish to be perfect, go, sell everything you possess and give to the poor, and you will have a treasure in heaven* (Mark 10:21 (NKJV)).

In keeping with the Trinity, he opened the Bible twice more, looking for confirmation. He saw: *Take nothing for your journey* (Luke 9:3), which was the command to the apostles, and: *If any man wishes to come after me, he must deny himself* (Matthew 16:24 (NKJV)).

Deny themselves they did, and soon the brotherhood swelled, welcoming people from all walks of life. Francis is known for preaching to everyone, including animals! One story has him preaching to hundreds of birds about how they should be thankful for everything that God has provided them, and that they sat intently until he finished, then flew away. Stories like that are the reason Francis is also the patron saint of animals and ecology.

As one Catholic resource puts it, "He did not try to abolish poverty, he tried to make it holy."[22]

When Francis wanted official approval for his growing brotherhood, he went to Pope Innocent III in person and was promptly thrown out of Rome for trying to approach the pope in his rags. That night Pope Innocent III had a dream about Francis in his poor attire holding a tilting basilica. When he woke, he called Francis back and approved his order.

Years later he relinquished control of his order that had swelled to five thousand in just ten years. His final years were filled with suffering, blindness, illness, and humiliation. During that time, he wrote his Canticle of the Sun. He ultimately is said to have received the stigmata, after praying to share in Christ's ultimate suffering.

He died at age forty-five.

At the time of Francis' death, he requested this reading:

Psalm 142
"I cry aloud to the Lord;
I lift up my voice to the Lord for mercy.
I pour out before him my complaint;
before him I tell my trouble.
When my spirit grows faint within me,
it is you who watch over my way.
In the path where I walk
people have hidden a snare for me."

My father was also influenced spiritually by the true story of Edgar Cayce. Cayce lived in the early twentieth century and used hypnosis to place himself into an altered state in which questions of healing could be asked, and answers would be given by angels

---

[22] Catholic Online, "St. Francis of Assisi," Catholic Online, Accessed November 13, 2021. https://www.catholic.org/saints/saint.php?saint_id=50.

through him. I highly recommend you read his exceptionally documented true-life story, *There Is a River: The Story of Edgar Cayce* by Thomas Sugrue.

Through his trances, Cayce prescribed treatments for a wide variety of medical maladies over decades. Each treatment was specific to the person and came from nature, supporting my father's belief that everything we need for healing is provided for us by God on Earth.

When Cayce was fourteen years old, he had just completed his fourteenth reading of the Bible when he said an angel appeared to him in his bedroom.

"She had said to him: 'Your prayers have been heard. Tell me what you would like most of all, so that I may give it to you.' He had answered, 'Most of all I would like to be helpful to others, and especially to children when they are sick.' Then she had disappeared and the next day she had helped him with his lessons."[23]

It wasn't until he was an adult that he discovered hypnosis, and under trance, was able to communicate and ask things of his angel.

Cayce passed on healing dictated from above, but his life was not without pain and suffering. He struggled to support his family and dealt with the derision of others. At one point, after many years of work and struggle, Cayce built and ran a healing hospital in North Carolina, only to have it go under during the Great Depression.

Among the Bible passages that helped Cayce take leaps of faith during difficult points in his life was this one:

Psalm 46

"God is our refuge and our strength, a very present
help in trouble.
Therefore we will not fear, though the earth be removed, and though the mountains be carried into

---

[23] Thomas Sugrue, *There Is a River: The Story of Edgar Cayce*, (Virginia Beach: ARE Press, 1997), 101.

the midst of the sea;
Though the waters thereof roar and be troubled,
though the mountains shake with swelling thereof.
Selah.
There is a river, the streams whereof will be made
glad the city of God."

Cayce left behind fourteen thousand psychic recordings but never once asked his angel about the nature of the universe or the soul, or about right and wrong, or the nature of all things. Cayce believed those questions to be sacrilegious, believing that God is revealed in the Bible, and to ask such things would have been an invitation for the Devil to speak through him. He stayed true always to his prayer as a child, to be an instrument to help others, particularly the sick.

Lorna Byrne

Someone whom I believe to be a living prophet on this earth right now is Irish mystic Lorna Byrne, who says she's been able to see and communicate with angels her entire life. Lorna is the international best-selling author of Angels in My Hair and a series of books about her interactions with and messages from the angels.

Among those messages is a prayer of healing she says was given to her by the Archangel Michael from God. This is that powerful healing prayer:

Prayer of Thy Healing Angels

Pour out Thy Healing Angels,
Thy Heavenly host upon me,
And upon those that I love,
Let me feel the beam of Thy Healing Angels upon
me,
The light of your healing hands.
I will let Thy Healing begin,

Whatever way God grants it,
Amen.

Lorna was very kind and graciously agreed to have a conversation with me for this book about the power of spiritual healing and dying with grace.

On the importance of faith when facing a terrible diagnosis, Lorna says, "Faith is important for everyone, not only when you are ill, but within every aspect of your life. By the sound of it, your da's faith even grew stronger, and that happens an awful lot when somebody is very ill. Their faith grows stronger because they go in search of God and their spirituality, their soul. They actually become closer, and sometimes—not all the time, but sometimes—God grants either extra time or healing for them in some enormous way that even doctors get puzzled by it.

"So I would always say when somebody is ill, everyone around them needs to have faith. It was just like with my husband; I asked for extra time for him and God gave the extra time, and it looks like God gave the extra time to your da. You were only nine, so you are not quite sure whether your da in his faith asked God for extra time so that you would be that bit older [when he died]."

I told Lorna about when my father was diagnosed, that I remember praying harder than I've prayed in my entire life.

Lorna said there was a big lesson to take from that, saying, "The faith of the child is, an awful lot of the time, billions of times stronger than an adult. Because an adult has been so conditioned by the world. So the faith of the child—it could have been God answering *you* more than your da, and it helped give him the best quality of life possible for those eight years."

Lorna says that may have been the miracle right there. She goes on: "I often would say there are millions of people standing in front of a firing squad and the bullets have already left; they are in slow motion.

"People get lost and terminally ill, lots of men, women, and children. Yet incredible miracles happen through faith at times, but not for everyone, and that is the hardest thing for everyone because everyone wants a miracle for their loved one when somebody is terminally ill or is going to die. There is a lifespan with them and the quality deteriorates, and it brings families together most of the time and helps family's faith to grow as well, and that is another miracle as well.

"Your da was about healing and changing his food. He was listening to his guardian angel to do everything to help his human body, and God granted him the extra time. Your da, in other words, chose his path in healing to put in the extra eight years."

I asked Lorna if part of faith is also accepting that His will is not always yours.

"Yes, that is correct, and people feel that they know that, and again that is another reason why their faith as well grows strong. They know it's not in their hands, and it is not actually in the hands of the doctors or in anything they do, but that it is completely in the hands of God, whether God is going to take you home to heaven or leave you here for a little longer.

"I know your da responded to everything he was told to do by his guardian angel and by God, and that is why he had the good food and maybe exercise, or you know, got the fresh air, sat by the sea. He was listening all the time. He was opening spiritually that he was healing so clearly, and I think that is wonderful; I call that a little bit of the intertwining of the body and soul, for the body to be able to stay a little bit longer."

Then I asked her to talk a little bit about one of her favorite topics: the incredible power of prayer.

"A prayer like praying as a child. You think of the child's words, think of the emotion. Prayer is extremely powerful; I tell people prayer can move mountains. People in the world today don't believe enough in prayer and they don't pray enough. I would say to all the things that are happening in the world, that if they all got together and prayed, if they can talk without saying, 'You're a different religion than I am so you cannot pray with me.' We are meant to [pray together].

"Prayer is prayer, and it does not matter whether you are a Muslim or if you are Catholic, a Protestant, a Hindu, or whether you are standing on your head or you are dancing in prayer. Prayer is prayer, and prayer is extremely powerful. It is one of the most powerful graces that we have been given to change everything, to change our hearts, and to change the world, and to allow healing to happen within not just the human body but our emotional self as well. To soften us. Prayer does everything; it increases our compassion and allows our understanding, it helps us to see hope in our lives, and I just wish people would pray, pray more.

"It was over the years people asking would I do a prayer book, and I eventually did, as you know, it is out now, and I always remember giving it to my publishers and him just saying this is not like an ordinary prayer book, this is a modern-day prayer book, and I loved that. I loved that he said it was a modern-day prayer book, and that is why I have to smile, but prayer is extremely powerful and I hope you are praying at times, and you can pray whether you are sitting on a bus; you do not have to be on your hands and knees.

"God knows the world has changed, but many people forget that. So God accepts prayer no matter whether you are here standing somewhere, traveling on a train, or just sitting on the plane. You can pray anywhere at all. There is no excuse not to pray. I think we use excuses all the time, even if there is loud music and your faith is music and playing, you can pray and that music or that loudness fades away.

"You know, I'm delighted your da put that book together with the amount they did and they are still going to benefit. What we want is for it to touch people's hearts for them to allow healing for themselves or for even the family that has someone that they become more conscious of all of the little lessons he has given within us, to, say, eat organic foods, pure food, good food and drinking clean water, having time and not rushing the way we do rush in the world today, to take time out to sit on the beach or sit by a river or sit under a tree—you know, things that people are doing nowadays. They are only doing those things sometimes, and they go on a holiday if they go on a holiday.

"He sounds like a good man. He was doing his best in life. Indeed, it sounds as if he achieved a huge amount. And in that part where he spent as much time with his children is a very important message as well. Your da is giving the message that even when you are not ill, you should spend more time with those you love."

For the record, I let Lorna know I pray most when I'm stuck in traffic.

Speaking of prayers, I asked her to share a few words about the Prayer of Thy Healing Angels that she shares in her memoir, *Angels in My Hair*. Lorna tells me those words are extremely powerful.

"The thing is, when Archangel Michael gave me that prayer, he carried the words of God, and when it was written down first, it was on a sheet of paper and it took ages. I do not know how Archangel Michael had the patience. But then my husband wrote it down on another few sheets of paper, and eventually it was put on a little card. After Joe had died and I had written the first book, *Angels in My Hair*, it went into that book."

She says that since the book was published, the prayer has gone worldwide in all different languages, and that it took considerable effort to make sure the words remained the same in every language.

She describes the words as the light of God. "God is using the healing angels, using that person when he stretches out and lays his hand upon them. It's an absolutely beautiful prayer. I am hearing from all around the world all the miracles that the prayer is connected with."

Lorna says it's not only a prayer of physical healing, but mental and spiritual healing as well. "It's everything. Sometimes when I'm giving a talk to someone, I say that prayer, and my anxiety is gone now."

But of course, Lorna is best known for her connection to the angels. According to her, every living person has a guardian angel who stays with you your entire life and never leaves your side. When you pray, Lorna says your guardian angel prays with you, but it can never interfere with your free will which God has given us.

Some of Lorna's books talk about ways to connect with your angels and feel them around you and grow that relationship. I asked her how people in a desperate situation can connect with the spiritual energy around them.

"When we do become ill, we kind of get afraid, so we reach out, we try and allow ourselves to become open and believe that there is more to life, and I think family and friends should help. I think people do help by giving them the prayer or saying the prayer with them. But then if someone has great faith, you know, that is no problem, the angels come in, in and around them, those healing angels, and the guardian angel is right there and he is holding on to them and filling them with support and strength that they need to be in this world for as long as they are meant to be, and there are so many things you could say, like when I go into a hospital or if I am walking down the street and I see someone that is terminally ill and nobody on the street would even notice. I would see sometimes the angels just come in and around him just for a brief moment and then leave. And then I would see the guardian angel just embracing them completely, and I believe that the person is given a zest for life to fight this illness. They get to understand how important it is, the wonderful gift that we have been given of life."

My father certainly had a zest for life, and faith, and lived far longer than he was supposed to, but it was not an easy journey. He was still very sick. He suffered from seizures and various other illnesses, and it was very difficult on me and my brothers. My brothers in particular had a lot of difficulties after he passed away. Lorna and I talked about how it's not always cut and dry. It's not always a pretty journey, even when you do get the miracle of extra time.

"You lived through every aspect of your father's illness, and that had a huge impact on you. Mentally, even physically, emotionally, and everything in that way, and at times you must have been mad with your da, and wishing that life was just ordinary like your friends down the street. Then other times, you know, you were scared, and you just wanted to love him, and you just didn't know whether you were coming or going. It is a very difficult time.

"My own children went through it, and they were the same, probably, as your brothers, or even as yourself. We kind of close out a lot of memories sometimes, and then something brings them back and it fills you with a little bit more love and compassion for others that are going through this at a certain stage in their life. Because even after my husband died—Joe—my children, who are adults now, found it very hard to go to a funeral; they did not want to do that because they felt they could not cope with it or visit someone that was seriously ill."

I responded that my brothers are exactly the same. It's sometimes difficult for people to understand why bad things happen. They want to know if they are being punished. They think, "Oh, God is not here. Why is this horrible thing happening to me?" But that is not right.

To that Lorna says, "No, you are not being punished. That's the question that is thrown at me all the time. Why is God punishing us? Why is this horrible thing happening? We were born to live and we are going to exit the human body. The human body is born to die.

"Most of the tragedy, separate from illness, happening in the world is caused by man. Man also causes an awful lot of diseases as well. God is not punishing you when your body gets sick, but we don't want to accept that the human body is frail; it's strong, but it's frail. It's like everything, it's open to disease, and even when you look around nature, you know, nature grows, it thrives, but then sometimes it gets a disease and something dies, or there is a fire, or things just grow to a certain age like flowers; sometimes it's just the summertime and then they wilt away. The same is true with everything of nature around us.

"But we find it very hard, because we want our loved ones to live forever. When we are facing the situation, we give out to God and say, 'Why is God doing this? Why is God allowing this horrific thing to happen? Why did God allow my child to be knocked down by a car and killed? Why did God allow my child to be raped, you know, or to be abused?' But God doesn't do it, it's man. We have the choice. We have the free will not to do these things."

Life goes on after death, Lorna says.

"It does. You do not die, because we have a soul, and I have written about it in all of the books, especially in *Angels at My Fingertips*. You have a soul that is that spark of the light of God, and it fills every single part of you. You don't die, you live, because your soul is immortal, it lives forever. It has everything about you, and even the soul of a loved one can be around someone, and they feel that presence, and sometimes somebody would say, 'I could smell my mom,' or 'I could smell the cigars my grandfather was smoking,' or the pipe, or something like that.

"Or sometimes somebody would say, they were just rooting through this drawer that they have rooted through for the last number of years, and just when they had been going through a hard time, they find this photograph or they find a feather and they cannot figure out how that got into that drawer, and then that can be a sign from your loved one, just letting you know that they love you and it will be okay.

"Our loved ones are all around us. They are fleeting; that's the word by the angels God has told me to use. We think sometimes that the soul of a loved one is in and around us twenty-four/seven, but it really is only a fleeting moment. But I am glad we feel that way.

"You know, I bet that you could feel the presence of your da around you. You are doing this book, so your da is definitely around you. You know he has inspired you, giving you the courage. He has probably been doing this and God has probably been allowing this to happen to give you the courage, and it has just been probably happening all of your life, and now you have the courage to do this, and you put it in the hands of God."

I told her I hope that I can put this book out there and that it helps someone.

"Well, then it's up to God, and this is up to the world as well. All you can do is put something out there and everyone else has to respond. Remember, even if only a few respond, or a huge number of people respond, if your book helps even one person—that is what I used to say with *Angels in My Hair*, if it helps even one person, that was my job done. It was to help someone, and that is the important thing, if it helps someone that happens to pick your book and read it, that is the important thing."

Finally, I asked Lorna about dying with grace when all of our times ultimately come. How can you make that passage easiest for yourself and the people around you?

"One thing I have written in the books that I tell everyone when it comes near your time to leave, you are filled with peace, complete peace, and your guardian angel takes hold of your soul and just brings the soul home, and at that very moment, your soul will see all those that have gone ahead of you and you are not afraid. It is peaceful.

"Sometimes the human body jumps and does things, but that has nothing to do with death, it's not the person suffering or anything like that, and lots of people think it is, but it is not. Everyone feels peace, and sometimes, someone won't let go because they feel their loved one around them and are not ready for them to go, but sometimes a loved one has to tell the person who is dying, 'It's okay, you can go now.' We have to let them go as well, because it is wrong for us to hold on to them and allow them to continue to suffer when there is no need, when they want to go. But lots of times we hold on to them ourselves, and sometimes a person will wait. Let's say a son or daughter was away and they are on their way back because they just got the news, and lots of times, you know that loved one will wait until that person arrives, and then just lets go and goes home to heaven.

"There is actually no pain whatsoever. I know sometimes even when someone thinks someone is suffering from pain, it's only the body; they are not actually really feeling it, you know, when they get to that stage."

And she tells me having faith makes everything easier.

"It does, it does. I have been asked since 2017—and this is 2018 now, started in 2017—and you know, priests, bishops, rabbis, ministers, nuns, you name those who are the heads of different faiths, different religions, and they are asking me one question, which I was very shocked, and that was, 'Is God real?' And I just look at them, astonished, because they study and they are meant to have faith.

"God is real and that is what we have to remember, and we have a soul. Your da is not dead. He is very much alive—so maybe the human body has died and decayed and turned into dust, but your da is alive and happy and at peace and so proud of you and your brothers.

"You put this into the hands of God, you don't put it into your hands, that is what your da did too. He put everything into the hands of God and he was given more time. He was blessed with more time even though it was really hard at times."

It's definitely not easy watching someone you love deteriorate, especially at a young age. That is why I resonated so much with Lorna's books, because she says she was warned her husband would be sick and die young even before she met him. That gave me a lot of peace in knowing that sometimes these things are just meant to happen.

My father's faith was strong, but so was his mental discipline and will to live.

Mental Fortitude

Oh boy. I'll be honest. When it came time to write this section on mental strength, I found myself feeling very weak.

How could I tell others to be strong when I had so much hurt and fear and grief on the inside, when I struggled to find focus and strength and self-discipline in my own life? I cannot even articulate why writing this was so hard for me.

I had a bit of a breakdown. I saw a therapist for the first time in my life to address the anxiety and depression I had battled alone my entire life. I took a break from writing, and at that time I had my beautiful daughter Desiree. I spent long nights while nursing thinking about what it was that I needed to say and how to say it. I always knew that I would finish. I had to. For me and Nicky and Desi and Ron, and my brothers and my mother and uncles, aunts, and cousins, and the strangers who desperately need to read these words and feel hope.

My father talked about visualization and other exercises that he believed helped him to boost his own body's ability to heal itself.

Before I get to that, I want to talk about my own experience with visualization and how it saved me during some of the hardest and scariest times in my life.

It was very traumatic having my happy little life turned upside at a young age. My father got sick when I was nine years old, and even though the initial surgery was a success and the tumor did not return for nearly three years, he did suffer from frequent, terrifying seizures. We three young kids were often left home alone with him while my mother worked long hours to keep the family afloat.

Out of nowhere, he'd suddenly drop, and we'd all have to jump on top of him to keep him from hurting himself. My job was to try to put a sock in his mouth (he bit through his tongue several times) and call 911 while my younger brothers held him down and cried. Sometimes he would stand up, while still totally unconscious, his black, lifeless eyes open as his body stumbled around the house while not registering anything we screamed. Afterward, he'd have no memory of it.

He began wearing a whistle and pill pack around his neck with his seizure medication. When he felt a seizure coming on, he'd blow the whistle so us kids would come running. Sometimes I'd be in a deep sleep when that whistle blew, and I'd wake up and my body was already running.

It was a lot to process, and we had no kind of direction or support. My mother had to work and no one sat us down to see what was happening emotionally with us, or guide us on how to deal with what was happening. The three of us suffered what I know now to be years of toxic stress.

By age ten, fear was my life. Not just fear of the next seizure, but fear of death, of dark spirits, of the dark, of spontaneous combustion, of aliens, of any number of things. The fear consumed me night and day. For my entire life until that point, I had slept with my whole family in one room. My parents, brothers, and I had the master bedroom, while my grandparents and my uncle occupied the other main rooms of the house. We also rented out a downstairs room for extra money.

When I was ten, my grandparents and uncle moved out and my parents asked the renter to leave. Suddenly my brothers and I all had our own rooms. I was too terrified to sleep in mine. I continued to sleep with my parents until one day, while I was still ten, they decided that the best way to end my fear was to cut me off cold turkey. They locked me out of the room. I remember screaming and shaking in the hallway, looking into my room, and thinking that it felt like a portal to hell. I cried all night, terrified to go in, only sleeping in the morning when the sun finally came up.

Over the course of several years, I barely slept. I could go days without sleep. I was exhausted, but my brain never stopped. I was tormented by dark and terrifying thoughts and unrelenting anxiety. Fear was not strong enough of a word. It felt like terror in my brain all the time.

Sometimes I would count red cars in the street to try to stop my brain from thinking horrible things, but it never fully worked. It finally got to the point when I was about twelve and a half that I started to wish I was dead. I wanted to die.

I share this story now only because I hope it will help others identify and help a child in crisis. There was one time when I was having a total breakdown—I forget what triggered it at the time but I was crying and shaking uncontrollably. I kept repeating, "I want to go home, I want to go home." My parents couldn't comfort me. They yelled at me that I was home and what was wrong with me. When I didn't stop repeating myself, they put me out on the porch to cry by myself until I calmed down. I needed to not be alone in that moment. I needed help.

I don't blame them though. They were frustrated and my father easily got headaches from noise. They didn't have the knowledge or tools to help with the emotional turmoil we were going through and they had my two younger brothers to manage also.

But, when I was saying that I wanted to go home, by "home" I meant heaven. I wanted to die. In essence, I was saying I wanted to die over and over again and I was left alone, to crawl back into the house and cry in my terrifying room the rest of the night.

It was about then that I started to want to hurt myself. It was that feeling of wanting to hurt myself that finally triggered something in me. That's when I remembered . . . I remembered being happy. I loved having fun and dancing and singing and watching movies and reading Harry Potter and going to Orlando theme parks with my family. I found pockets of respite at school, where a few hours at a time my brain would stop terrorizing me and I'd laugh with friends, or go to a school dance. I wanted more of that.

I didn't want to die, I wanted to be happy again. As someone later said so eloquently, I wanted my circumstances to die, not me.

My mental suffering also manifested into night terrors, sleep paralysis, and sleepwalking. I apparently would have these episodes where, if someone disturbed me while I was sleeping, my body would shoot up and start yelling, "Who are you? What do you want?" etc. I never remembered these episodes, even though sometimes I was yelling quite loudly. These events continued well into my thirties, which I believe was some kind of PTSD response to what I went through as a kid. My husband learned to ignore me and tell me to go back to sleep. He wasn't amused when I punched him one time.

Anyways, as I said, my parents were thoroughly occupied and not equipped to help me. They didn't know what was wrong with me or how to address it. I think they hoped I would just grow out of it. Plus, it wasn't a family in which anyone talked about their feelings, ever, even about this. On the contrary, we kids were discouraged from talking about all my father's seizures while he was left home alone with us because it made him feel bad to hear how scared we were.

When I reached out to counselors at my middle school for help, they called my parents and told them I had violent tendencies (I did not) and didn't listen to what I had to say and didn't provide any support that could help me. I was not referred for therapy and no interventions of any kind came of it. This was the same time that Columbine happened, so I think the schools were too busy looking for threats to see where they should be helping instead. I had no adults to turn to. Those few friends who made me happy at school weren't enough to solve what I was going through.

I had to turn within. I had to save myself.

At nearly thirteen years old, I finally told myself that one day in the future I was going to look back at all the things that used to scare me and I was going to laugh.

It wasn't long before that became a reality.

I did it using visualization.

At night, when I was most tortured and terrified and couldn't sleep, I started to imagine myself inside a little bubble of light.

At first, this bubble was weak, but inside of it, I could rest my weary mind for a few minutes at a time. I visualized filling the bubble with light and pushing all the dark and terrifying things to the outside. I prayed that God would help me.

Little by little, that bubble grew stronger and brighter! I felt safe in my head for longer periods of time as I worked every day and night on making the bubble stronger in my mind. I filled my bubble with my happiest memories and feelings. Pretty soon I felt like laughing! I pictured myself inside my glowing-white bubble laughing at all the terrible things on the outside while I was surrounded by light and joy on the inside. Sometimes visualizing the cross made it even stronger. The more I practiced focusing on my bubble, the stronger it became and the longer I could keep my mind there.

Soon I was sleeping through the night in my own room! At first, it was with the light on and the TV blaring. Then with the TV on but the volume turned down. Then with the light switched off, which was *huge* for me. I kept pushing myself to get better. I wanted to win!

During the day I popped in and out of my mental bubble when I needed it. I focused on school the best I could, although my public middle school was poor and full of gangs and drugs. My family couldn't afford to keep sending us to private school anymore after my dad got sick, so we all ended up in public.

My family moved to a better neighborhood when I was fourteen. That meant a better school! And I kept fighting for that happiness of mine. It was never given to me, being happy and making the best of my circumstances, rising above and setting myself up for a good future; those are all things I fought for and did for myself, without exterior help. I fell into TV production and newspaper and stayed after school every day learning the craft of truth-telling.

That's where I began my career in journalism.

So let's take a deeper dive into visualization and how it can unlock some of the hidden power of your awesome brain!

If there is no enemy within, the enemy outside can do us no harm.

—African proverb

The power of the mind cannot be understated. You may have heard of Tibetan monks who can raise their body temperatures by using a certain kind of yoga meditation. It has been thoroughly documented, and using solely the power of their minds they can raise their body temperatures up to seventeen degrees in their hands!

Research affirms that we can effect dramatic changes in our own bodies by simply willing it to be!

Dr. Clifford N. Lazarus in *Psychology Today* writes, "Visualization and imagery techniques are not medically recognized as first-line treatments for cancers or for most any serious diseases but as adjunctive therapies, they can be very helpful. Indeed, as I'm fond of saying, 'The mind and the body are different sides of the same coin and they intersect most strongly at the level of imagination.'

"In fact," he continues, "the brain and the nervous system weave into all the tissues of the body and affect them in very important ways. And because of the two-way street that connects the mind and psychology with physiology and biology, the mind itself can affect the body in many powerful ways."[24]

I think we've only barely scraped the surface of what man is capable of. There are many resources out there that can help hone the power of your incredible mind from *The Secret* to yoga to world religions to hypnosis or simple psychology that can re-frame your world and set you on the path to success. My father made beating his brain tumor his ultimate path of success.

Human consciousness is real and the interconnectedness of the

---

[24] Clifford N. Lazarus, "Can Visualization Techniques Treat Serious Diseases? The Amazing Power of the Mind-Body Connection and Psychoneuroimmunology (PNI)." *Psychology Today*, January 26, 2016. https://www.psychologytoday.com/us/blog/think-well/201601/can-visualization-techniques-treat-serious-diseases.

mind and body are profound. Many studies have shown that focused thought can demonstrably have an impact on the physical, both positive and negative.

A great book to read in this vein is *The Biology of Belief: Unleashing the Power of Consciousness, Matter & Miracles* by Bruce H. Lipton, PhD. In it, Dr. Lipton writes, "We are not victims of our genes, but masters of our fates, able to create lives overflowing with peace, happiness, and love."

Dr. Lipton argues that "gene activity can change on a daily basis. If the perception in your mind is reflected in the chemistry of your body, and if your nervous system reads and interprets the environment and then controls the blood's chemistry, then you can literally change the fate of your cells by altering your thoughts."

This supports the overwhelming evidence that negative thoughts and stress can create a damaging inflammation response in the body that can cause or exacerbate any number of ailments and diseases. Meanwhile, the power of a positive attitude, while more difficult to quantify, has been shown to boost the body's immune response and decrease damage from stress hormones.

Anger is an acid that can do more harm to the vessel in which it is stored than to anything on which it is poured.
—Mark Twain

A resource from Johns Hopkins Medicine titled "The Power of Positive Thinking" shares that, "The mechanism for the connection between health and positivity remains murky, but researchers suspect that people who are more positive may be better protected against the inflammatory damage of stress. Another possibility is that hope and positivity help people make better health and life decisions and focus more on long-term goals. Studies also find that negative emotions can weaken immune response."

It goes on to say, "What *is* clear, however, is that there is definitely a strong link between 'positivity' and health. Additional studies have found that a positive attitude improves outcomes and life satisfaction across a spectrum of conditions—including traumatic brain injury, *stroke*, and brain tumors."[25]

Another researcher, Dr. Kelly Turner, explains it this way in her book *Radical Remission*: "Neuropeptides that have a healthy effect on your immune system include serotonin, dopamine, and relaxin; these are released whenever you feel relaxed and happy. Neuropeptides that have a weakening effect on your immune system, especially over an extended period of time, include cortisol, epinephrine, and adrenaline; these are known as stress hormones. What makes stress—or any emotion, for that matter—so powerful is that almost every cell in our bodies has the ability to both produce and receive these neuropeptides."[26]

Dr. Turner has written two very important books, *Radical Remission* and *Radical Hope*, in which she spent decades investigating hundreds of stories like my father's, people who refused to die, and against all odds, were cured or went into "spontaneous remissions" that were scientifically unexplainable. She aggregated the things that most of these super-survivors have in common and begged the question, why was nobody studying them?

Among the commonalities she found among these extraordinary people were "Radically changing your diet; Taking control of your health; Following your intuition; Using herbs and supplements; Releasing repressed emotions; Increasing positive emotions; Embracing social support; Deepening your spiritual connection; and having strong reasons for living."[27]

Dr. Turner has also launched the Radical Remission Project where others can share their stories of miraculous survival or where you can read the inspiring true stories of many others. I've

[25] "The Power of Positive Thinking." *The American Journal of Nursing* 86, no. 2 (1986): 118–19. https://doi.org/10.1097/00000446-198602000-00004.

[26] Kelly A. Turner, *Radical Remission: Surviving Cancer against All Odds*, (San Francisco: HarperOne, 2014).

[27] Ibid.

submitted my father's story to be part of the Radical Remission Project.

Another person who forged their own treatment and recovery by using the power of positive thinking was magazine editor Norman Cousins. In 1964 he was diagnosed with a life-threatening autoimmune disease and given a one in five hundred chance of survival. From the very beginning, just like my father, Cousins rejected his diagnosis and instead created for himself a regimen of happiness. Literally, laughter became his best medicine.

This happy therapy included regularly watching Marx Brothers films, and he credited it for his dramatic recovery. Similarly, my father talks about how he scheduled regular massages for himself and made relaxation and enjoyment a part of his routine when he could. Not to mention my father's unwavering faith gave him peace and joy. Medical science in the '60s and '70s scoffed at the idea that any emotion, positive or negative, could have an impact on the course of a disease or on the body. But studies conducted in the 1980s and early 1990s would reveal that the brain is in fact directly wired to the immune system.

Cousins went on to found the Norman Cousins Center for Psychoneuroimmunology at UCLA, which is "dedicated to investigating whether psychological factors really can keep people healthy."[28] They are partnered with the Mindful Awareness Research Center at UCLA, whose mission is to "disseminate mindful awareness across the lifespan through education and research."[29] There are resources, research, audiobooks, free guided meditations, and more that you can access through their organizations' web pages.

Conversely, repetitive negative thoughts have been shown to

[28] "Cousins Center for Psychoneuroimmunology at the Semel Institute for Neuroscience and Human Behavior," UCLA.edu. Accessed January 14, 2022. https://www.semel.ucla.edu/cousins.

[29] "UCLA Mindful Awareness Research Center, Los Angeles, CA." UCLAHealth.org. Accessed January 14, 2022. https://www.uclahealth.org/marc/.

significantly contribute to stress and disease in the body. Stress puts the person into a survival state, which exhausts the body and not only causes physical harm, but adverse responses like depression, anxiety, anger, misery, and confusion. The neurochemicals produced by these things can be highly addictive and people can become trapped in these cycles of negativity. Maybe you've noticed yourself or people in your lives who are seemingly addicted to drama or seem to make the same mistakes over and over again.

The brain needs to be redirected, and with the power of will and intentionality, a person can reprogram themselves to achieve whatever they want. But it takes hard work and repetition, certainly, in my experience.

Another interesting researcher worth learning about is American psychologist and parapsychologist Dr. William G. Braud, who dedicated his career to the study of human consciousness. Dr. Braud put his findings together in a book called *Distant Mental Influence: Its Contributions to Science, Healing, and Human Interactions.* In it he details ways in which we can not only mentally influence our own bodies through techniques like visualization, hypnosis, intention, and other forms of self-regulation but how those techniques can be used to foster physical and psychological health and well-being in subjects outside of ourselves.

Dr. Braud details decades of meticulous research that purports to show that such techniques can be used at a distance for the purposes of healing, that these abilities can extend to animals and even human red blood cells, and that his findings could support the efficacy of distant, mental, or spiritual healing and intercessory prayer.

Dr. Braud published more than 290 papers in his lifetime, including peer-reviewed articles and three books. I highly recommend reading some of it as his findings are absolutely fascinating.

My takeaway is this: You have awesome power. Use it.

"I can't," you say. Stop it. You can. The only one limiting yourself is *you*.

Focus on your intent, practice if you have to, and stay consistent.

The power of the mind is great, but I believe that the power of Him is greatest. We're only just scratching the surface on what human consciousness is and where it resides in the brain. Some of the latest research, of the quantum variety, suggests consciousness could exist independently of the body and that the mind is merely a vessel or conduit for a consciousness that goes on even after death. There is no doubt in my mind that that is the soul and that we are on this earth to grow and learn, and that no matter how small we believe ourselves to be, our purpose is big and important. We have been given the power to shape this beautiful world around us, and unlocking the power of our consciousness (i.e., soul) and of our minds to influence the world around us is something the human race needs to open itself up to more.

I want to hear more stories like my father's. I want to hear about people taking control of their circumstances and breaking all the rules, bending the rules of what we know to be true, and making those supposed barriers submit to their awesome God-given will.

I tell my son that God gave us free will, and that believe it or not, the power to choose really is a superpower. I believe that wholeheartedly.

Tips to Realign Your Mind

First and foremost, help yourself clean house of mental gunk to help yourself be more receptive to realigning your mentality. What helped me the most was knowing that I was not alone.

YOU ARE NOT ALONE. There is energy outside of ourselves. Call it God, call it the greater universe; I think that power is all one and the same. Open yourself to the possibilities, allow yourself to receive. Give yourself permission to find peace and healing. Find support where it is good and true. Now is a good time to reach out to helpful people—friends, family, and support groups. Find those people who feed you with positivity and remember that you are important.

YOU DON'T DESERVE TO SUFFER. Many times we feel that we must suffer. Subconsciously our insecurities, fears, traumas, and regrets tear us apart and set us on a painful path. Take some time to sit down and think about where certain feelings come from and give yourself permission to let them go.

Sometimes we go through terrible experiences and we feel guilty or undeserving. As my friend Dwight once said, if we didn't have the bad we couldn't identify the good, and how much better it can be. Sometimes we need a positive person in our lives to realize that we do deserve to be happy. Let me tell you, *you deserve to be happy*. Today is the day that you are alive, you can make your own happiness, don't punish yourself anymore, let the positivity in, let it grow, water it, and nurture yourself.

PRACTICE SELF-AWARENESS. This is essential to cleaning house, as it were, of the muck that sometimes holds us back. When you feel something, practice pausing and thinking about where it comes from and what you can do about it. Practicing self-aware-ness clears the field to allow more positive energy into your mind and into your life in general. It can also help prevent destructive behavior. Seeing a therapist who respects your goals and your challenges can also be a great help.

BE CONFIDENT IN YOUR GOODNESS. This was a big one for me, especially since I feel like I've always been terrified of dark energies, or fearful that my good intentions could be motivated by selfishness or other guilt-inducing things. Let your love shine through. We were all born as pure love, and various difficulties and traumas of life cause us to block out that love and form negative behaviors or self-beliefs. Take time out of every day to find that love within yourself and nurture it to grow. This can be pretty scary, but love is the energetic key to healing, I believe. Love yourself more. Challenge the walls you've built around your heart. Believe in your goodness; don't look to others to give that to you.

FORGIVE YOURSELF AND OTHERS. Don't let anger, resentment, or hatred (self-hatred or otherwise) hold you back. Those emotions own you; they control you and keep you from moving forward. They accomplish nothing but feeding darkness, stress, and degeneration within you. Don't let negative feelings own you. When you forgive, it is a triumph. Those feelings no longer have a stranglehold on your mind, and it makes room for the positivity that you're going to need to heal yourself. That is to say that you shouldn't just allow toxic people in your life; you can forgive *and* distance yourself or remove toxic individuals or situations in your life. These are not mutually exclusive. You'll need a good team of positive people around you.

BE OPEN-MINDED. Many times we get swept up by the material, superficial world around us, the need for money, and the hustle of life. We get disconnected from our interior world and the possibilities of life and the universe that we can manifest ourselves. Take a step back and open yourself to the possibility that there is more to life than what lies on the surface. Not every technique is going to speak to you, but keep trying until you find what can help you change the world around you.

LAUGH A LOT. Watch that funny movie, spend time with your loved ones, play with the kids, look at funny memes. Laughter is the best medicine! Science can prove it! Movies and books have played a big part in my happiness in this life (*Star Wars!*). Those feel-good brain chemicals can only help you find peace and positivity.

DON'T GIVE UP! As Winston Churchill once said, "Never, never, never, never, never, never give up!"

Now that we've swept away some of the mental junk holding us back, there are plenty of visualization techniques that can be helpful depending on what works best for you. Everyone is different! From guided meditations, hypnosis, psychotherapy, yoga techniques, or a visualization of your own creation, explore robustly! My father talks about how he took time every day to focus on imagining that he was zapping his own tumors with a ray gun and making them disappear. When I was terrified and couldn't sleep or stop my negative thoughts, I built a little ball of light around myself in my mind. I worked tirelessly day and night to make that ball of light stronger and brighter until I finally felt safe in my head again.

Do the research, put in the work, and find what works for you! You are worth it!

Mental Health

All of this is not to say that if you struggle with your mental health, you are failing. FAR FROM IT! You wouldn't be human if something like this wasn't completely traumatic. Build your medical team, support network, and bring a professional psychotherapist into the mix, if even only occasionally. Caregivers, you need to care for yourselves as well. I really truly wish my family would have done this, but the pervasive attitude back then was that seeing a shrink meant you were crazy. There was a very negative stigma around struggling with mental health. Add the fact that my family talked about *nothing*, and I feel there were a lot of mental agonies we suffered that were just totally unnecessary. In the cases of my brothers and me, there were underlying issues that exacerbated our trauma as well, like ADHD, ADD, anxiety, and depression. It wasn't until we were adults in our thirties that these issues began being addressed.

A great organization to connect with is Imerman Angels. They provide free one-on-one support by connecting patients and caregivers with others going through the same experiences. Seek out organizations like this one.

Talk! Talk to a trusted professional, a friend, your spouse, or a fish, it doesn't matter. Talking helps you to process, ease fear, and move forward. Not to say that it will be a straight line. I'll admit that I had at least two full-blown mental breakdowns while writing this book, because reliving what we went through with my father being sick most of my childhood was very difficult for me. But I never gave up. I finally got help and picked myself back up and kept going. That's all we can hope to do. My advice is to prioritize your self-care and your mental well-being along with everything else.

Need Motivation?

Stop making excuses for why it's all over. *Fight*. Don't defeat yourself! Can you do it? Of course you can. Believe in yourself, and the world around you will change. Claim your power; no one else can give it to you. If it helps to have someone else believe in you first, know that I believe in you!

Fear is fake. Don't be afraid of pain. Pain is what's necessary to make a transformation. Or as the United States Marine Corps puts it, "Pain is just weakness leaving your body."

> *Destiny is not a matter of chance, it is a matter of choice; it is not something to be waited for, it is something to be achieved.*
>
> —William Jennings Bryan

Death is coming for us all, so in the meantime, why not try to change the fabric of the universe around you using your mind, body, and soul?

Listening to the best of Queen always puts me in the mind

frame for conquering the world. What gets you in the mood to fight the good fight? What pumps you up?

Unger Motivation on social media is a great place to find some inspiration and hope. He is a cancer survivor as well and an ultra-athlete.

Find a local running group; in my experience, they are a great place to find super supportive people.

I also did aikido for many years while I was an award-winning news producer for CBS Radio in Washington, DC. My sensei was a cancer survivor named Michael Veltri. He was a great inspiration to me, and he also has a book called *The Mushin Way to Peak Performance: The Path to Productivity, Balance, and Success.*

Michael was a thirty-something Marine veteran, martial arts master, and corporate wunderkind, working full time during the day and operating an aikido dojo at two small locations in Washington, DC, by night when he found a lump in his testicle. He thought he was a textbook case of early detection, surgery, and remission. He had low cancer markers after his surgery, and for the next three months, he had regular CAT scans and bloodwork to ensure the cancer was gone for good. That's when, while feeling confident that he could move on with his life, he walked into his doctor's office and was told bluntly, "The cancer has spread to your lungs. We need to start chemo immediately."

Michael said he felt like he had been hit over the head with a two-by-four. But he was oddly relieved that it hadn't spread to more devastating areas. He felt it was game on.

But while most patients might do chemo once or twice a week, Michael told me his doctors recommended six hours a day, five days a week, for three unrelenting months. The aggressive course of treatment destroyed the new tumor, but it also took a tremendous toll on him both physically and mentally. Chemotherapy kills not only the dangerous cells but destroys many healthy cells along the way as well.

Michael tearfully recounted the pain he suffered, the agonizing sores he developed in his mouth, and his inability to move or eat.

His doctors ultimately recommended surgery to remove the remnants of the tumor from his lung, which left him without a lower left lobe of his lung and in a wheelchair.

All of this was naturally a grievous challenge to someone as strong-willed and self-reliant as Michael. But it wasn't long before he fought his way back.

He tells me he found that the most important things to have when facing a devastating diagnosis are twofold: people and things.

"You'll need positive and supportive people who you can call or lean on when you're feeling your lowest," Michael said. He adds it was difficult, especially as a man, to let himself be vulnerable and rely on others, but says it was incredibly important to get him through the worst moments. Just to be able to pick up the phone and call a friend and say, "Today is really hard, this really sucks," helped him tremendously.

He really needed his buddies there to make fun of him, make him laugh, and lift him up. His mother also dropped everything to take care of her son, something he's eternally grateful to have had.

The "things" part is things that pick you up and make you happy. He found a lot of relief and solace in watching feel-good movies and reading books. As a matter of fact, Michael Veltri used to be one of the biggest Harry Potter haters around (when he mentioned this, I jokingly threatened to cut off the interview and our friendship), but he says while doing chemo he picked up the first Harry Potter book just to have something to do and was instantly hooked. Those books provided the same fun, inspiration, and escape that they provided me when dealing with my father's illness. Sometimes you need to lose yourself in a story about wizards and dragons defeating evil to get through the hardest times. His friends also bought him a portable DVD player so he could watch funny movies wherever he went. Other days he'd spend the day at the dojo in his wheelchair on the sidelines just surrounded by the people and things he loved.

These are also all a part of what he calls the Four S's: Support Structures Sufficient for your Success.

"Where your focus goes, your energy flows," Michael told me. "If all you do is focus on the negative, then you'll absolutely find a million negative things and you'll be stuck there. But if you focus on the positive, your energy is going to go there and you are going to see incredible things that you never knew existed."

It can be difficult, though, in the throes of your darkest hours.

"I always tried to find the light," Michael told me, "because there are times that there is nothing but darkness around you." He always tried to bring those bits of light around himself by focusing on them and enveloping himself in them, much like my visualization story.

Michael also made a point about fear and facing your own mortality.

"It wasn't that I wasn't afraid. I was. Everyone is. It's just like a saying we had in the marines. Everyone is afraid before going into combat. If they say they aren't, they're lying. What is important is to recognize the fear and not let it control you."

Michael often shares this perspective when asked: "Once you survive cancer or anything that is life-threatening, everything else is easy. It's all about perspective."

Michael has since moved on from teaching martial arts and is now a best-selling author and inspirational keynote speaker.

Seize every moment to make the most of life, that's what I learned from Michael Veltri. Case in point, I just happened to have been on a trip to Japan with my dojo on my twenty-sixth birthday. Our generous hosts had given me several birthday cakes that I couldn't possibly finish, so Michael and a few students and I ended up in a small bar on the island of Okinawa with one of the cakes. I said I wanted to share it, so Michael seized the moment. He talked to the bar man, who announced to the whole place that I was sharing my cake with them. A dozen strangers proceeded to cheer and sing happy birthday to me in Japanese and broken English. It was one of the coolest and happiest moments of my entire life. That's the energy you're going for right there!

Again, physical activity is a great way to get yourself motivated and promote healing in your body, from running to yoga to mountain climbing. Get your body moving! The American Cancer Society confirms that patients who exercise regularly and maintain a healthy diet heal better and remain healthy longer.

Which leads me to the final aspect of my father's self-treatment that I believe played a major role in his longevity.

Nutrition

Mind and body go hand in hand. From exercise to nutrition, how we care for our bodies can make all the difference between a death sentence and a miracle.

My father considered his regime to be a nutritional approach to cancer treatment. It was difficult for him, after subsisting on junk food all his life, to suddenly upend his entire diet, but he did it. I remember him dragging us to meetings with nutritionists and dietitians and one lady who invited us to her home to teach him how to use a juicer.

There are fabulous books available out there today that can help you begin to conquer your cancer through nutrition! I recommend reading *Chris Beat Cancer* by Chris Wark, a long-term survivor of stage III colon cancer. In 2003, at twenty-six years old, Wark was diagnosed with stage III colon cancer that had spread to his lymph nodes and had a golf ball–sized tumor growing in his large intestine. He rejected chemotherapy, just like my father had done when he was given no hope for survival with his brain tumor. Chris, instead, transformed his diet to a super healthful one and tried every natural, nontoxic treatment he could.

All these years later, he's not only alive and well but thriving!

In his book, Wark credits the core of his anti-cancer strategy to "consuming 15–20 servings of organic fruits and vegetables per day by *juicing*, eating my *giant cancer-fighting salad*, and drinking my *anti-cancer fruit smoothie.*"[30] His book is a great read on how to superpower your immune system to attack your cancer, and how faith and nature combined to bring him back to health. Chris offers health and coaching on his website as well and has a very helpful and inspirational blog.

There are many other great reads out there, including *Beating Cancer with Nutrition* by Dr. Patrick Quillin, *Stop Feeding Your Cancer* by Dr. John Kelly, and *How Not to Die* by Dr. Michael Greger. I list some of the great resources in this arena at the back of this book.

Here's the added challenge, though: Many drugs, cancer and seizure medications included, can have negative side effects. You can't always avoid these realities. My father relied on his seizure medication, which made him bloated, prevented him from losing weight, and was hard on his liver. Other forms of cancer respond well to certain traditional treatments that have negative side effects on the body like painful tissue damage, inflammation, lowered immune system, loss of appetite, exhaustion, and weight loss. So doing everything you can to give your body the good fuel it will need to fight off disease, boost the immune system, and heal from treatment is imperative.

In fact, poor habits can actually *cause* cancer. According to the American Cancer Society, "At least 18% of all cancers and about 16% of cancer deaths in the US are related to excess body weight, physical inactivity, alcohol consumption, and/or poor nutrition."[31]

Sometimes the foods we love the most could be doing us the most harm. The World Health Organization has classified processed meats (think bacon, hot dogs, and processed lunch meat)

---

[30] Chris Wark, "Anti-Angiogenesis: Foods That Fight Cancer," Chris Beat Cancer, July 12, 2010. https://www.chrisbeatcancer.com/anti-angiogenesis-cancer-fighting-foods/.

[31] Cheryl L. Rock et al, "American Cancer Society Guideline for Diet and Physical Activity for Cancer Prevention." *CA: A Cancer Journal for Clinicians* 70, no. 4 (2020): 245–71. https://doi.org/10.3322/caac.21591.

as a Group 1 carcinogen, meaning "there is convincing evidence that the agent causes cancer," in particular colorectal cancer. Similarly, the WHO has classified red meat as a Group 2A carcinogen, meaning the connection is not as clearly observed in studies, but there are strong associations between eating red meat and developing colorectal cancer.[32]

Keep in mind that your mainstream doctors, including general practitioners, are not required to take *any* credit hours on nutrition in medical school, so there seems to be a blind spot many times where doctors ought to be linking diet and disease.

For those who are already sick, the American Cancer Society has great data, research, and tips on maintaining good exercise and nutrition during and after cancer treatment, along with other free resources on their website.

They've published a cookbook called *What to Eat during Cancer Treatment* with more than 130 recipes, as well as practical tips to help patients eat well during treatment.

It is imperative that you make an appointment with a board-certified specialist in oncology nutrition to aid you through the duration of your treatment. A naturopathic cancer specialist can also help guide you in the direction of not only a healthy diet, but toward the many natural supplements, herbs, teas, etc. which have proven anti-cancer properties. Shark cartilage is considered a dietary supplement, and my father details everything he took in the herbs and supplements index at the back of this book.

The American Cancer Society has positive things to say about diets rich in antioxidants like blueberries, chia seeds, cruciferous veggies, garlic, and green teas. These superfoods may also support anti-angiogenesis, which is the slowing or stopping the formation of blood vessels that feed tumors. This is the same effect

---

[32] "Cancer: Carcinogenicity of the Consumption of Red Meat and Processed Meat," World Health Organization, October 26, 2015. https://www.who.int/news-room/questions-and-answers/item/cancer-carcinogenicity-of-the-consumption-of-red-meat-and-processed-meat.

that shark cartilage is purported to produce. Eating multiple servings of fruit and vegetables per day is a great way to reduce your
risk of diet-related diseases, and many, including my father,
achieved that intake by juicing.

Other foods like flaxseed have anti-cancer properties to help
support cancer patients during and after treatment. The reason
flaxseed meal, in particular, has so many health benefits, besides
being packed with nutrients and omega-3 fatty acids, is because
of its strength as a dietary fiber.

One tablespoon of whole flaxseeds contains three grams of
fiber, which is around ten percent of the daily recommended
intake. Not only does it promote gut health and healthy bowel
movements but the flaxseed binds to bile salts that are then ex-
creted by the body. Your body pulls cholesterol from your blood
into the liver to replenish the bile salts, lowering your blood levels
of cholesterol.[33]

Flaxseed is also a great natural source of lignans, a plant com-
pound with antioxidant and estrogen properties that can lower
the risk of certain cancers. Four out of five breast cancers are fed
by an imbalance of estrogen.

By removing excess hormones from the body, fiber can be
considered one of the most protective nutrients in the fight against
cancer. According to the Physicians Committee for Responsible
Medicine, "In the United States, the average daily fiber intake is
10–20 grams per day, but experts recommend at least 30–40 grams
per day. The best sources of fiber are minimally processed whole
grains, beans, peas, lentils, vegetables, and fruits. Foods that are
closest to their natural state, unrefined and unpeeled, are highest
in fiber."[34]

---

[33] Mette Kristensen et al.,"Flaxseed Dietary Fibers Lower Cholesterol and
Increase Fecal Fat Excretion, but Magnitude of Effect Depend on Food Type."
Nutrition & Metabolism 9, no. 1 (2012): 8. https://doi.org/10.1186/1743-7075-9-8.

[34] Kerrie K. Saunders, *The Vegan Diet as Chronic Disease Prevention: Evidence
Supporting the New Four Food Groups.* (New York: Lantern Books, 2003), 199.

Fiber also helps prevent cancer by drawing water into the digestive tract, making stool bulkier and softer, helping to flush carcinogens from your system while minimizing their contact with the walls of your intestines.

Too Much Information time! Let me tell you that I have struggled with constipation since I was a child. Nothing in my life that I have tried (and I've tried stool softeners, olive oil—you name it) has made me as regular and cleaned me out quite as well as flaxseed meal. I'd love to shout from the rooftops how just one tablespoon a day has already improved the quality of my life.

But I digress.

There is great literature out there about starving cancer with the power of a healthy, packed diet. Again, see my list of recommended reading at the end of this book.

Always discuss your use of herbs, supplements, and other natural remedies with your oncological team—in particular, that oncology nutrition specialist or naturopathic cancer specialist. Seek out the specialists.

It is not recommended to self-medicate with natural remedies without the supervision of a medical professional, as some herbs and supplements can have negative effects. For example, Essiac tea is touted as an alternative cancer treatment. Lab studies suggest Essiac has antioxidant and cytotoxic properties; however, according to the Memorial Sloan Kettering Cancer Center, "Studies on its antiproliferative effects are conflicting: Essiac prevented the growth of prostate cancer cells but stimulated the growth of breast cancer cells. In a study of breast cancer patients, Essiac did not improve quality of life or mood. Despite unsubstantiated claims, Essiac remains a popular anticancer therapy."[35, 36]

My father also had a negative experience while taking a DHEA

---

[35] Kristen S. Kulp et al., "Essiac and Flor-Essence Herbal Tonics Stimulate the in Vitro Growth of Human Breast Cancer Cells," *Breast Cancer Research and Treatment* 98, no. 3 (2006): 249–59. https://doi.org/10.1007/s10549-005-9156-x.

[36] Barrie Cassileth, "Essiac," *Oncology* 25, no. 11 (Williston Park: 2011): 1098–99. https://www.mskcc.org/cancer-care/integrative-medicine/herbs/essiac.

supplement. He details experiencing sudden amnesia while taking DHEA in the herb and supplement index at the back of this book.

My father had to seek the outside advice of Dr. Dante Ruccio when it came to managing his intake of shark cartilage and balancing it with the other supplements he was taking. His oncology team at the time was strictly against anything but the standard chemo and radiation protocols.

It does seem, however, that there have been great strides in the last two decades of incorporating integrative medicine into some mainstream cancer treatment, so that is very positive for those fighting cancer today.

Another inspirational person who is worth following, and also happens to be a personal friend of mine, is weight-loss champion Chuck Carroll. He overcame food addiction and dropped from 420 pounds to 140 pounds without going to the gym! You can find him and his incredible story on his website TheWeightlossChampion.com or hear him host the podcast *The Exam Room*, put together by the Physicians Committee for Responsible Medicine.

A common topic on *The Exam Room* is how diet and lifestyle can play an enormous role in whether you develop certain cancers, or how your eating and exercise habits can help you heal from or prevent disease.

Case in point, Carroll on *The Exam Room* got to share the remarkable story of Kate McGoey-Smith. You can find her podcast interview on *The Exam Room* from August 24, 2021, entitled "Whole Foods Plant-Based Diet Saved Her Life." Carroll told me, "[She] was given two to five years to live after being diagnosed with a rare disease. This was over ten years ago! She's healthier than ever today. As a bonus, she reversed diabetes!"

McGoey-Smith reversed blindness, reversed type II diabetes (she had a 15.1 A1C), and is fighting rare idiopathic pulmonary arterial hypertension, a terminal disease that is essentially localized high blood pressure in the pulmonary arteries in the lungs.

She suffered severe symptoms including shortness of breath,

swelling, quick depletion of oxygen, and severe right-sided heart failure.

It took nine months to get her diagnosis in 2007, and while taking medications and experimental drugs given to her by her doctors, McGoey-Smith lost her eyesight and her kidneys were so damaged that she's been in end-stage kidney failure since 2013.

While blind, hooked up to oxygen, and listening to television, she heard about a book called *Dr. Neal Barnard's Program for Reversing Diabetes: The Scientifically Proven System for Reversing Diabetes without Drugs.* After hearing Dr. Barnard speak in person and appreciating the science behind his nutritional approach, she and her husband decided to make a radical change to the way they ate.

She now credits a plant-based diet with keeping her off dialysis, restoring her eyesight, and bringing her body back to health, allowing her to fight her terminal diagnosis effectively by slowing the progression of the disease.

Chuck Carroll also interviewed the next mayor of New York City, Eric Adams, who said in a November 13, 2019, *The Exam Room* episode that he, too, used a plant-based diet to regain his eyesight and reverse diabetes. Adams details his story in the book *Healthy at Last: A Plant-Based Approach to Preventing and Reversing Diabetes and Other Chronic Illnesses.*

Carroll told me that some of the doctors he's spoken with are big on using nutrition as the first line of defense for preventing diseases. He recently interviewed Dr. Kristi Funk, who is a breast cancer surgeon in Los Angeles. Her client list includes Angelina Jolie and Sheryl Crow. On an October 19, 2021, episode of *The Exam Room* titled "Top Anti-Estrogen Foods with Dr. Kristi Funk," she told Chuck that she believes as much as ninety percent of breast cancer cases are preventable and that estrogen plays a huge role, calling estrogen "breast cancer candy."

Dr. Funk says one way or another, she makes sure she and her sons eat these three foods every single day to balance the natural production of hormones in the body and prevent cancer: soy, cruciferous vegetables, and flaxseed.

We've talked about cruciferous veggies and flaxseed, but soy is a very healthful and helpful food as well. The American Cancer Society says, "There is growing evidence that eating traditional soy foods such as tofu, tempeh, edamame, miso, and soy milk may lower the risk of breast cancer, especially among Asian women."[37]

Chuck Carroll is a warrior, a health cheerleader, and a strong plant-based nutrition advocate who is often joined on his podcast by Dr. Neal Barnard, researcher and author of the book on using nutrition to reverse type II diabetes. Please check them out.

I also had a great conversation with a naturopathic cancer doctor, Ian Bier, ND, PhD, LAc, FABNO. Together we talked about taking a whole-body approach to cancer treatment.

Dr. Bier says he got into naturopathic medicine back in the 1980s when he himself was a patient. "I had no desire to be a conventional doctor. Basically, I had all sorts of health problems on my own that conventional medicine could not help me with at all, mostly gastrointestinal, and eventually, they literally gave me my chart and said, 'Check yourself into Hopkins, we do not know what is going on.'

"I was diagnosed with celiac back when it was not even called celiac and the head of gastroenterology in the hospital had to look it up in a textbook. But, basically, a friend of my mother's told us about this naturopath—quacko-path-type as I called it at the time—in Toronto, which is three hundred miles away, and she needed someone to drive her there. So I drove her there and saw him myself and he told me what was going on with my body and gave me changes in diet, supplements, and treatment. Then lo and behold, I got better, and so that is how I became interested in medicine."

---

[37] Stacy Simon, "Soy and Cancer Risk: Our Expert's Advice," American Cancer Society, April 29, 2019. https://www.cancer.org/latest-news/soy-and-cancer-risk-our-experts-advice.html.

Dr. Bier says oncology became his specialty because many cancer patients started to come into his clinic and he wanted to treat them the best that he could. He eventually became a fellow of the American Board of Naturopathic Oncologists and became a naturopathic oncologist specialist.

Many people may not even be aware that such specialists exist, so I asked Dr. Bier how precisely a naturopathic cancer specialist can help.

"Number one," he says, "and you may already know this, the American Association of Naturopathic Physicians is like the AMA of conventional doctors, and they have a good website with information on the profession and what the education is like and comparing the number of hours in accredited schools to conventional medical school, etc. So they are a great resource for that. The Oncology Association of Naturopathic Physicians, ONC-ANP, is the professional organization for the oncologists, and again they have a website and they have all sorts of information, you know, all the materials that could give you the kind of background for a larger perspective than just mine.

"My background is research and statistics, so I say to people, I wear two hats. My love is the prevention and treatment of cancer with diet, supplements, and treatment, which we spend a lot of time on, and also I am a big proponent of what I am terming; I kind of dropped holistic and alternative and conventional and western and integrated and all of those wonderful terms and I really talk about informed medicine."

Dr. Bier says he tells patients who are interviewing him that he is like a financial planner, but with oncology. "They have to figure out how to rebalance their portfolio, their risks, and benefits, where they are putting their intention, and the only way to do that is to know real information.

"How effective is what is being offered to them conventionally, if anything, for their particular condition? This is the most important decision-making process and journey of people's lives and we need to have the appropriate information to make that decision. Are we talking about ninety-five percent or five percent cure or remission rate with conventional therapy?

"There are literally therapies that are ninety-five or more percent survival rate, and there are literally ones that are zero, no change in lifespan at all, but also have some side effects."

Dr. Bier has this advice for patients who are ever faced with a physician who comes to them with absolutes (for example, you absolutely must do chemo or you're going to die, or you must absolutely never do chemo): "They are just a demagogue and not paying attention to the unique individual and what their situation is.

"All of my patients, if they want me to, I serve that role of financial or informed consent advisor and we look at it and dig out the research and we find the best information we can and we say, oh, look this clinical trial. This sounds like a bad joke, but it's real: Two men walk into the doctor's [office] within a month of each other, both have head and neck cancer, which is getting more and more common. The first gentleman has already had surgery and now it's back. They take a look at it and they want to do radiation therapy on him, put him in a mask every single day for I don't how long. He cannot swallow, they may have to put a feeding tube in, and the difference in chances of survival over five or ten years is a couple of percentage points. He decides not to.

"Next gentleman comes in. He's got a very similar case but he is HPV positive; the same virus that contributes to cervical cancer, right, far more aggressive cancer because of the virus. I pulled the paper, I looked at it, I looked at it again, I blinked. At ten years, ninety-five percent of people are still alive if they do the radiation; it is a much more aggressive cancer, but it responds to the radiation incredibly well because it is virally driven.

"Of course, that is a totally different scenario, right? The end of the story is he still chose not to do it. He felt good about what we were doing. He thought he was going to be fine. I was like, 'So you are clear you understand what I am telling you, right? Repeat it back to me, if you will.'

"'Yes, I understand, if I do the radiation my chances of surviving ten years is about ninety-five percent, it's as close to cured as you can get.'

"'Okay, good, you still don't want to do it?'

"'I don't want to do it.'

"'Okay, then my job is to help you.' So it's really to be responsible about it; it is helping every single person look at their situation. Breast cancer in a forty-year-old, for example, is a different disease than breast cancer in a seventy-year-old."

As far as a smooth working relationship between traditional oncologists and naturopathic specialists, Dr. Bier says it is often a crapshoot. "I am on the board right now for the naturopathic oncologists; we are having discussions about residency training in a new practice area. One of the things we talk about is doing rotations with conventional doctors to see what it's like. People on the West Coast are like, 'I have great relationships with this oncologist and it is not a problem, and of course you should do it.' For me here on the East Coast and some of my colleagues up in Canada, it's like, you've got to be kidding. They are ten years behind. They do not even talk to us.

"I did have a wonderful conversation with an oncologist two weeks ago, and then I have had people where they are like, if you are doing any of this stuff I won't treat you, and kick [the patient] out. So it's completely variable. There is a wholesale change that needs to happen, where we all need to learn that we are service providers and we work for the boss, and that boss is the patient. They get to make the decisions. But that is slow in coming, I think."

We talked about how it's important to find a provider who will honor your wishes and take the time to know you and your circumstances. It's not recommended to self-medicate without a doctor's guidance and monitoring, whether that be a conventional doctor or naturopathic one or, preferably, both who can work together. It certainly can be difficult, but it's important to build that solid, supportive team around you.

I asked Dr. Bier whether he's anecdotally seen better outcomes when people use either holistic or complementary treatments along with traditional therapies.

"I think my patients do far better than predicted, better than they expected. You know when you are dealing with cancer that has been treated, is in remission, and has a statistical chance of coming back, you know, someone who underwent a lumpectomy or a mastectomy, somebody that had part of colon removed, someone who did radiation therapy, it is really easy to go, 'See, it never came back,' instead of going, 'Okay, there was only always a ten, twenty, fifty-nine percent chance of coming back.'

"When you are dealing with a stage IV patient who statistically has zero chance of survival to their regular lifespan, I do not think anybody is getting miracles. Do better than predicted? Yes. Better quality of life? That I am comfortable with. I would say that my [stage IV] patients tend to be functional far longer, and then when they do start to transition, it tends to happen very quickly, which is a blessing.

"There is ample data that what we do has potential for a very positive effect. Unfortunately, with the internet and with everybody's hopes, it kind of ends up being just, 'Well, is this a cure?' 'Can I go down to Mexico and cure this?' and the fact is that there is no cure."

Which brought our conversation to my father's particular story. I explained to Dr. Bier how my father, Jimmy Blanco, was diagnosed in 1995 with a glioblastoma multiforme grade IV, given three months to live, and he chose not to do chemo, not to do radiation, none of that. He instead started taking shark cartilage, which at the time was emerging and popular. I explained how he also transformed himself nutritionally and how he utilized methods of visualization, hypnosis, and his intense faith to try to heal himself.

I explained how my father began writing this book to document his journey, and part of that journey involved encountering the snake oil salesmen out there and how the first shark cartilage he purchased was useless injectable sugar water. Later, a book called *The Cure for All Cancers* landed him in the hospital.

I asked Dr. Bier how people should do their due diligence when encountered with an extraordinary story like my father's. It's certainly never been proven that the shark cartilage was primarily responsible for him living eight years after his diagnosis; however, when somebody hears a story like that, what do they want to be cautious about? I don't believe that the shark cartilage was the only thing that helped him, although he attributed his longevity most especially to that. So what advice does he have for people who hear these stories and you want them to pause and get all the answers before they decide to take a radical self-treatment?

"I think there are a couple of aspects. One, I am talking to you as the primary source who was there with your father. That's rare. Most of the time it's somebody who heard something from a friend who knows somebody else that it happened to. In today's world on the internet, people lie, right, they just straight out, flat out lie. So that is the problem. And then with a stage IV glioblastoma, there is no question there, living eight years is a miracle versus the 'I had breast cancer and did Essiac tea and it went away,' and then you trace it down, it's like, 'I had a low-level lesion that may not have been breast cancer/ductal carcinoma *in situ*, I did lumpectomy, radiation, and Essiac, I just did not tell you.'

"Then, I think the other piece of it is miracles happen, if you want to define a miracle. I generally say a miracle is you wake up one day and it is gone. Anything less is really good results. But eight years quite fits on that level. But the key is, is it consistent? Miracles don't come from me, I tell patients. Miracles don't come from curcumin and shark cartilage, miracles come from wherever you believe miracles come from. You tell me that you went down to Mexico and cancer went away and you got documentation, and even I see the documentation, that is awesome, except I know people who went to Mexico and had to be medevacked back."

Dr. Bier laments that people who don't do conventional treatment drop out of the system and are not tracked by medical science.

Conclusion

This book is a memory of a miracle. Both my
father's and mine.
It is a testimonial, and I hope it inspires you to
have the courage to seek out answers, to defy
convention, and find peace within yourself, as we
all must ultimately go home at the end of this life.
If this book helps just one person, I will have
accomplished my goal.
Godspeed, and God bless you.

Index of Herbs
and Supplements Used

by Jimmy Blanco

810-ZYME

Suggested to me by Dr. Ruccio. I had been taking other enzymes, but I decided to stick to this one. Enzymes play a huge role in just about all body activities. They are essential for maintaining the proper function of the body, digesting food, and aiding in the repair of tissue. The body manufactures its own supply of enzymes, but it can also obtain enzymes from food. Unfortunately, low degrees of heat will destroy enzymes in food, so in order to obtain enzymes from the diet, the food must be eaten raw. Those who do not eat raw foods or supplement their diet with enzymes put an undue strain on the supply of enzymes in their body. Enzymes are apparently the only nutrients that can supply the body with the energy needed for its activities, so overuse, according to what I've read, can impair the body, making it susceptible to cancer, obesity, cardiovascular disease, and a host of other illnesses. Trypsin and chymotrypsin are examples of proteolytic enzymes. These enzymes are extracted from unripe papaya and pineapple.

ADVANCED ANTIOXIDANT FORMULA

This comes in the Cambridge label. Recommended by Dr. Ruccio, I give this product credit for cleaning my blood. During the course of my treatment, I had my blood checked under a microscope, and the doctor was surprised to find such a low number of free radicals on a cancer patient. Antioxidants help protect our bodies from the formation of free radicals. Free radicals are atoms that can cause damage to our cells, which in turn impairs our immune system and can lead to infections or disease. If your diet is inadequate or lacking the appropriate antioxidant, look for a formula that includes the following supplements to aid the body in destroying free radicals: vitamins A, C, E, GLA, L-cysteine, L-glutathione, selenium, and superoxide dismutase (SOD). This formula is not the only antioxidant that I took, but I felt it was the best.

AGED GARLIC EXTRACT

Garlic is known as a natural antibiotic. It has been used since biblical times. Pyramid builders were apparently fed garlic every day to give them endurance and strength. Garlic lowers the blood pressure through the actions of one of its components, methyl allyl trisulfide, which dilates vessel walls. Garlic thins the blood by inhibiting platelet aggression, and this reduces the risk of blood clots and aids in the prevention of heart attacks. It also lowers cerium cholesterol levels and aids in digestion. Garlic is used for many diseases and illnesses, including cancer. In the beginning, I took any garlic pill, which was all right, but later I discovered that an aged garlic extract with enzyme was the best, and it is also odorless. I took two pills twice a day.

ALOE VERA

Aloe vera is a plant that I grew up with. My father would always talk about the healing powers of this plant. I never listened, because kids always know more than their parents, right? I would brush him off and tell him to leave me alone with that garbage. Until, finally, I discovered that my father was right all those years. You were right, Dad; I should have listened. In *Heinerman's Encyclopedia of Healing Herbs & Spices* by John Heinerman, he writes that when Columbus set sail for America, he wrote in his diary, "All is well, aloe is on board!" Aloe was the material used to embalm Pharaoh Ramses II and to preserve the body of Jesus Christ.

In *A Holistic Protocol for the Immune System* by Scott J. Gregory, he writes, "For over five thousand years, folk medicine has celebrated the juice of the aloe vera plant for its unique healing properties." Aloe vera contains six antiseptic agents. It's an anti-inflammatory and contains plant sterols, which are important fatty acids, including HCL cholesterol, campesterol, and B-sitosterol. Gregory writes, "These compounds also aid in allergies, arthritis, rheumatic fever, both internal and external ulcers, and inflammation of the digestive system. The stomach, small intestine, liver, kidneys, and pancreas can all benefit from these anti-inflammatory effects. Aloe not only provides vigorous overall immune system support but aids directly in the destruction of intra-vascular bacteria. The reason is aloe's unique polysaccharide component. The body's natural 'complement system'—a critical defense system involving a series of proteins—only needs to be activated in order to attack bacteria. It is the polysaccharides that trigger these proteins in a sequence called the 'cascade phenomenon'—to take on a doughnut shape and insert themselves into the surface membranes of bacteria. Through this action they literally create holes in the bacteria, exposing the pathogens' interior to surrounding fluids, causing their death."[38]

I stayed away from all the aloe vera products in the health food stores. The reason being I felt that this plant was too important to leave the processing in someone else's hands. The most natural thing you can do is to go to your supermarket and actually buy the aloe vera leaf yourself. My mother makes it quite enjoyable to drink. My mother is the aloe vera–making expert; I always let her do it for me. She takes the leaf and washes it first with water, then peels the outside portion and removes the insides. She places it in a strainer and rinses off some, not all, of the gelatin substance of

[38] Scott J. Gregory, *A Holistic Protocol for the Immune System,* 5th ed., Palm Desert: Progressive Press, 1993.

the aloe. After this is done, then she places it into a blender and adds bottled water, three or four whole lemons, and some brown sugar. Then she blends it for several minutes.

You can make it to your own taste by adding more lemons or more brown sugar. In the end, it tastes like a good lemonade. Aloe vera really has no taste, so it's easy to drink. Place it in the refrigerator; it tastes even better cold. I drank three eight-ounce cups a day. I felt as though my intestines and kidneys were getting a tune-up. It cleaned my insides well and kept me regular.

ARGININE

Arginine has ammonia reduction effects. I took one a day.

ASTRAGALUS

Astragalus is an herb also recommended by Dr. Ruccio. Using *Prescription for Nutritional Healing* by James Balch as a reference, I discovered the following: astragalus acts as a tonic to protect the immune system, as a diuretic to reduce edema (especially in nephritis), and as an anhidrotic. It aids the adrenal gland's function and digestion, increases metabolism, promotes healing, and provides energy to combat fatigue. I took two pills twice a day with meals for seven months. Now I take it in cycles, one month on and one month off.

BLACK WALNUT HULL TINCTURE

This herb is one of three herbs that were meant to be taken together to kill parasites. I took this because I read Hulda Regehr Clark's book *The Cure for All Cancers*. As I have mentioned before, I was not interested in who was right or wrong when it comes to cancer treatments. I was desperate and willing to try anything and everything as long as it gave me hope of surviving. The Black Walnut Hull Tincture is supposed to kill the adult and developmental stages of a hundred parasites. The parasite I was targeting was the human intestinal fluke (*Fasciolopsis buski*). The theory was that this parasite could cause cancers. I took one drop (qid) four times a day and added one drop a day until I reached twelve drops. At that point, I had to stop because I was hospitalized. I did not take this again after that.

BLESSED THISTLE

There were several reasons I added this herb to my treatment. First, it increases appetite, and I had lost thirty-five pounds due to poor appetite. Second, it heals the liver, which I needed to be strong to combat my cancer and process all these pills. It improves circulation, purifies the blood, and may act as brain food. *Warning:* Handle carefully to avoid toxic skin effects. I took two pills twice a day with meals.

CAT'S CLAW

Cat's claw (una de gato), or uncaria tomentosa, is the bark of a famous tree in the Peruvian Amazon. It's been used for many years for cancer. I received my cat's claw from someone that brought it directly from Peru. When that shipment finished, I stopped taking it because of rumors that one cannot be sure what they were getting in those capsules. I took one pill bid, or twice a day.

CHICKWEED

This herb is said to be useful against tumors and cancer. I added this one on my own also. I took two pills twice a day with meals.

CLOVES

According to the book *The Cure for All Cancers*, cloves kill the eggs of parasites inside the human body. I took one pill three times a day before meals. I increased by one until I reached three pills, three times a day, from day three through ten. Then I took three per day for the next two days until I stopped because I was hospitalized. I did not take this again after that.

COQ-10, 120 MG

Coenzyme Q-10 120 mg was recommended by Dr. Ruccio. I used the book *Prescription for Nutritional Healing* as a reference. This plays a crucial role in the effectiveness of the immune system. It declines with age and should be supplemented in the diet. In Japan, it is used in the treatment of heart disease and high blood pressure and is used to enhance the immune system. It claims that coenzyme Q-10 is a major step forward in the prevention and control of cancer. No side effects have been documented to date. It improves cellular oxygenation, increases circulation, and improves breathing. Aids in healing and is a powerful antioxidant. It is a powerful free radical scavenger.

DAILY FIBER

Even though I was getting fiber in the Earth Source Green, I took an additional fiber pill for a period of time. This is because I felt good elimination was essential for my recovery. I took three pills twice a day after meals.

DAILY MULTIVITAMIN

I took a high-potency, antioxidant-rich formula. I started with one brand that required two pills twice a day on an empty stomach for four months before I switched to another brand.

DHEA

I had a special blood test done to check my DHEA levels and the results came back very low. My levels were equivalent to that of an eighty-seven-year-old, and far from the normal for a thirty-eight-year-old man. I was told that in order to get well I needed to bring my levels up to normal. A local doctor recommended it to me (not Dr. Ruccio), so I started to take DHEA. Within two to three days, I stopped after I suffered a terrible bout of momentary amnesia. I was in a department store with my family. They were eating, and I decided to get up and go find something that I needed. As I walked through the store, I suddenly forgot what I was looking for. As I continued, I began forgetting where I was.

The more I walked, the worse the amnesia got. I suddenly forgot who I was and what I was doing there in this store. Panic began to set in; I was at the point where I was about to start screaming in the middle of this store. As suddenly as the amnesia came, it wore off when I saw my wife walking toward me. This was the worst experience I could have had. I felt as though I did not exist. I attributed this experience to the DHEA because I never had this happen before, and the DHEA was the only new supplement that I added to my program. Once I stopped taking it, it never happened again. I believe for one reason or another this hormone affected my brain. I do not recommend DHEA for anyone with a brain tumor.

ECHINACEA

Recommended by Dr. Ruccio, I took this herb two pills, three times a day. Echinacea is good for colic, colds, flu, infection, and snake bites. It has antibiotic, antiviral, and anti-inflammatory properties. Good for the immune system, lymphatic system, and glandular swelling. I took this on an empty stomach.

EARTH SOURCE GREENS & MORE

This is a unique blend of nature's most potent plant foods. It was also recommended by Dr. Ruccio.

ESTER-C POWDER WITH BIOFLAVONOID COMPLEX

Recommended by Dr. Ruccio, it's a vitamin C supplement. Bioflavonoids are sometimes referred to as vitamin P. Bioflavonoids reportedly enhance the absorption of vitamin C and they are beneficial when taken together. The human body apparently cannot produce bioflavonoids; instead, they come from the diet. Bioflavonoids have an antibacterial effect and promote circulation, stimulate bile production, lower cholesterol levels, and treat and prevent cataracts.

I drank one teaspoon of Ester-C with eight ounces of bottled water and half a lemon three times a day (TIO).

FENUGREEK

Fenugreek helps lower cholesterol levels. When I entered the hospital, my cholesterol level was very high. I began taking fenugreek and my levels are down close to normal. Cholesterol levels should be below 200; my level dropped to 206. I took two pills, twice a day. I stopped taking this herb and my levels are up again.

FLAXSEED OIL

Flaxseed oil was recommended by Dr. Ruccio. It is high in lignan and is certified one hundred percent organic. The bottle states it contains the richest vegetable source of omega-3. Lignan is a well-researched plant fiber found in the highest concentration in flaxseed. The brand I use must be refrigerated. I mixed a quarter cup of nonfat cottage cheese with two tablespoons of flaxseed oil once a day.

According to the American Cancer Society, "In the lab, flaxseed (and compounds from flaxseed) seems to have slowed cancer cell growth and helped certain treatments work better. In 2 small studies, patients with breast or prostate cancer who were put on a flaxseed-rich diet before surgery had lower rates of cancer cell growth (in their tumors) than the patients on other diets. More research is still needed to see the effect of flaxseed on outcomes."[39]

GENISTEIN PLUS

This has the Alternatives for Health and Healing label. Genistein Plus is composed of isoflavones, a type of phytoestrogen found in soybeans. The important isoflavones, genistein, and daidzein are being investigated for their wide-ranging health effects on the body. The formulation also contains L-glutamine as an antioxidant and to potentiate the activity of soy isoflavones.

---

[39] Cheryl L. Rock et al., "American Cancer Society Guideline for Diet and Physical Activity for Cancer Prevention," *CA: A Cancer Journal for Clinicians* 70, no. 4 (2020): 245–71. https://doi.org/10.3322/caac.21591.

GINKGO BILOBA

I added this herb on my own. I researched all the herbs and I added anything that would improve brain function. Ginkgo biloba improves memory loss, which I had a lot of. It also improves brain function, depression, cerebral and peripheral circulation, oxygenation, and blood flow. I took one pill a day with meals.

GINSENG & BEE POLLEN

I took this on my own. Ginseng is used throughout Asia to treat general weakness and give extra energy. If there was one thing I needed after surgery, it was energy. Russian scientists claim the ginseng root stimulates both physical and mental activity. Researchers suggest they also protect against the harmful effects of radiation. The hypoglycemic should avoid using large amounts of ginseng. The Russian approach is the most advised: use ginseng for fifteen to twenty days, followed by a rest period of two weeks. I recommend avoiding long-term usage of high amounts of ginseng, even though studies have shown no side effects. I used it only for a few weeks. I also expected it to stimulate my appetite and normalize my blood pressure. After I began my treatment, my blood pressure, which was high for the past fifteen years, suddenly dropped to normal and has stayed normal ever since. Many of the herbs I take are responsible for that. Bee pollen is effective for combating fatigue, depression, and cancer.

Warning: Some people may be allergic to bee pollen. Bee pollen contains the B-complex vitamins, vitamin C, amino acids, polyunsaturated fatty acids, enzymes, carotene, calcium, copper, iron, magnesium, potassium, manganese, sodium, and protein. Bee pollen, bee propolis, and honey have an antimicrobial effect. I took one pill a day for a few weeks and then discontinued them.

IMMUNOFIN

Immunofin is a naturally processed G-E lipids/alkylglycerols from pure shark liver oil. I took one pill twice a day on an empty stomach.

L-ORNITHINE

I took two pills at bedtime to help me sleep better. Ornithine is an amino acid that assists in the urea cycle. Parasites produce large amounts of ammonia as their waste product. Ammonia is very toxic, especially to the brain. The brain lacks the enzyme ornithine carbamoyltransferase, essential for making ammonia harmless by changing it to urea. This may have been the reason I was hospitalized. This might work better for other types of cancers. Brain cancer might not work as well. I did not know that this release of ammonia by dead parasites might be toxic to the brain.

LECITHIN

Lecithin is another group of chemicals needed by every cell in the human body. Cell membranes are largely composed of lecithin, and without it, cell membranes would harden, not allowing nutrients to pass through. The protective sheaths surrounding the brain are also composed of lecithin. This was the main reason I began taking lecithin. I was already taking lecithin in the Earth Source Greens & More, but I took an extra thousand milligrams twice a day by itself for a period of time. The Earth Source Greens has two thousand milligrams of lecithin. Lecithin helps prevent arteriosclerosis, protects against cardiovascular disease, and increases brain function. Lecithin is also known to promote energy and is needed to help repair the damage to the liver caused by alcoholism. Lecithin allows fats like cholesterol to be dispersed in water removed from the body.

MEGA-ZYME

Mega-zyme is an enzyme. I took this for about four months, then switched to another brand

MILK THISTLE

Milk thistle is an herb that I started to take because I was worried about keeping my liver healthy. I began to worry because I was experiencing pain in my liver area. I did research on the liver and discovered that the liver is our body's filter. It filters every-thing we eat, drink, and breathe. I did a chemistry profile and my GGT—which is an indication of liver function—was high. Normal is 0–64. My GGT was 155. Milk thistle is good for disorders such as jaundice and hepatitis. It contains very potent liver-protecting substances.

Silymarin is a standard milk thistle extract containing eighty percent (120 mg per capsule) silymarin, a flavonoid complex. Turmeric, a common spice, had been added to the product for its complementary effects. I started taking only one a day because I wasn't familiar with it. I later increased my dose to two pills, three times a day with meals. After a few weeks of doing this, I repeated bloodwork and my GGT had decreased to 62. After sixteen months I stopped all pills for one month. I continued the shark cartilage and the milk thistle. I did this to give my liver a break.

PARSLEY LEAF
Parsley leaf is a sweet plant that contains a substance that in-hibits the multiplication of tumor cells. I added this on my own and took three pills twice a day.

PHYTAID
Phytaid has a combination of herbs that are known to do well against cancer. It's supposedly an improved version of Essiac. In-gredients: astragalus root, Self-heal, echinacea, sheep sorrel, slippery elm, Indian rhubarb. It's not to be taken within one hour of eating. That means nothing to eat one hour before or after taking the Phytaid. One ounce of powder will make one liter of Phytaid. I drank three ounces three times a day. I took this for only one month. I found it very difficult to brew, but well worth taking.

RECOVERY POWDER DRINK
This anabolic recovery and nutrition drink was recom-mended by Dr. Ruccio. The brand I used is a very good-tasting

chocolate or vanilla drink. It claims to be a complete food that combines metabolic optimizers with the essential nutrients for rapid gains in muscle size, strength, speed, and stamina. I lost thirty-five pounds after my diagnosis. Many cancer patients lose weight and muscle mass and are generally weak. I think Dr. Ruccio wanted me to take this product to gain my strength back and stop losing weight. I drank the chocolate flavor. I had half a scoop mixed with bottled water and a spoonful of brown sugar once a day. I found it to be quite pleasurable. It tastes like a chocolate shake.

SUPERFOOD POWDERED DRINK MIX

I drank a powdered superfood drink mix on my own. The brand I used is a highly concentrated natural source of chlorophyll, amino acid, vitamins and minerals, carotene, and enzymes. It is a unique combination of barley, wheatgrasses, kelp, and the green algae chlorella. The barley and wheatgrasses are organically grown. Chlorella is a rich natural source of vitamin A, and kelp supplies iodine and other valuable minerals.

Any health food store will have it. I drank an eight-ounce glass three times a day. One of the main reasons I began drinking this product is because of all the literature I have read about wheatgrass helping cancer patients. Wheatgrass is a nutritional food discovered by Dr. Ann Wigmore. She claims that wheatgrass contains the greatest variety of vitamins, minerals, and trace elements, and that fifteen pounds of fresh wheatgrass is equal in nutritional value to three hundred fifty pounds of the choicest vegetables. Dr. Wigmore also reports that wheatgrass therapy, along with "living foods," has helped to eliminate cancerous growths and helped many other disorders, including mental health problems.

TEA TREE OIL

This has nothing to do with cancer, but I felt it was worth mentioning.

The 100 percent pure Australian tea tree oil is one of the most incredible natural products that I have come across. My wife, Elizabeth, was constantly complaining to me about an open cut on her hand that would not heal. She types all day as a medical transcriptionist and this was really bothering her. I did some research and I found the tea tree oil in *A Holistic Protocol for The Immune System* by Scott J. Gregory.

In it he states, "For centuries, the aborigines have gathered the leaves of this tree to rub on their skin, to heal wounds and cuts, and other skin ailments."[40] Its usefulness and properties include antiseptic, antimicrobial, antibacterial, antifungal, and mildly anesthetic. It is for wound-healing, cuts, scratches, abrasions, burns, sunburns, insect bites, scalds, allergic and itchy dermatoses, lesions caused by herpes, impetigo contagiosa, furunculosis, psoriasis, ringworms, boils, pimples, and an antiseptic essential oil for aromatherapy.

I bought it and used only the dipstick to run a very small amount across Elizabeth's cut that would not heal before she went to sleep. In the morning it was completely healed, just like that. I have also used it on my son Jimmy Jr. for his sinusitis. I rub a little across his forehead and a little down the side of his nose and it cleared up his nasal passageway. I have used it over and over on all my children, and it is incredible how well it works. I think it's a must-have in every home, especially if you have kids.

VITAL VEGGIES

This was recommended by Dr. Ruccio. For me they were very important because I never ate vegetables. I took one pill twice a day on an empty stomach. Some of the pills I took on an empty stomach because most of the other pills were specifically meant to be taken with a meal. I tried to not take too many pills at the same time by separating them so they all may be absorbed properly. I ordered this through Alternatives for Health and Healing. Each

---

[40] Scott J. Gregory, *A Holistic Protocol for the Immune System*, 5th ed., Palm Desert: Progressive Press, 1993.

capsule contains one hundred percent farm-fresh cruciferous veg-etables with beta-carotene. Vital Veggies are recommended for those who have poor eating habits, for people who do not enjoy eating these vegetables, and because cruciferous vegetables are not available year-round. Each capsule can be opened and added to soups, salads, and other foods.

WORMWOOD CAPSULE

Wormwood is from the artemisia shrub. It also kills adults and the developmental stages of at least one hundred parasites. I started with one pill a day and increased it by one every day until I was taking twelve pills a day. At that point, I stopped because I was hospitalized. I never took them again.

Letters

In this section, Jimmy shares a number of letters, as he wrote them. You will read letters written to the church on the occasion of his baptism into the Church of Christ, a letter to President Bill Clinton, and a letter he wrote to his insurance company at the time, AvMed.

Letter to the Church

The following was a letter addressed and read to my congregation at Sunset Church of Christ one month after my surgery and diagnosis.

One Man's Struggle with Cancer

I heard the three speakers the Sunday before Thanksgiving and I said to myself, "Who could be more thankful to the Lord than me?" I would first like to thank the Lord for allowing me to be here. I represent two miracles—going on three. I would also like to thank all the people that have prayed for me, many I didn't even know.

Special thanks to Mr. and Mrs. Ligon, Mrs. Prekins, and the entire Tropical Christian School staff for all the food and kindness they have given me and my family. I have never met nicer people in my whole life. I feel God has blessed me. Some people would have been angry with the cards God has dealt. I could have asked the Lord why He gave me a seizure on one of the happiest days of the year for me—my wife's and mother's birthday. I like to find the blessing in every problem, so I think it happened to show me miracle number one.

I had my seizure while driving to work with oncoming traffic. I was only a few blocks away from the hospital where I work when suddenly I was blind, deaf, and shaking violently. In less than five seconds I was unconscious. That's when the Lord took control of the wheel and guided me to a soft crash with a parked car in front of a house. I was awakened an hour later, and to my amazement, I was alive.

Police and fire rescue took me to the hospital, where a CAT scan and MRI showed I had a brain tumor the size of a baseball, seven centimeters. I needed to have it removed immediately.

They prepared me for brain surgery. With twelve years' experience in the medical field, I knew I didn't hit the lottery with this problem. I signed a living will and told my family I loved them and prayed that God wouldn't leave my three small children fatherless. I did not expect to come out of surgery alive.

Miracle number two: not only did I come out of surgery alive but I'm here with you today. After surgery, the doctors dropped even a bigger bombshell on me. They told me I was diagnosed with an (astrocytoma) glioblastoma multiforme grade IV—the worst and most aggressive type of brain tumor. They couldn't remove it all. They told me I am terminal with no hope of a cure. Doctors told me I have to do chemotherapy and radiation treatments. If I don't, I have three months to live, and even if I do, it will only prolong my life from six months to one year. Well, I never did have much faith in doctors. I put all my faith in the Lord. I believe that prayers help more than any of the doctors' treatments. Only God can tell me when my mission on earth is finished. I refused all of their treatments along with their side effects.

All the doctors have counted me out, but I feel that my mission on earth is just beginning with miracle number three. The Lord will heal me and I will be a testimonial that will inspire many others. God could heal me on the spot if He wishes to.

Sometimes He will guide you in the right direction so that in healing you, you in return could help others be healed without traditional therapies. This experience changed the way I look at life. It's a shame that it took this traumatic event to bring me closer to the Lord. There are some things I have learned and am inspired to share with everyone:

1. When you see someone full of hatred, treat them with love.
2. Find the blessings in every problem.
3. Don't hate anyone. We are all brothers and sisters and universally intertwined.
4. Spend as much time with your family as possible. We don't know how long we have to enjoy them.
5. Always give when someone is in need without expecting anything in return.
6. If you think negatively, your health will suffer. So always think positively.
7. Life will always provide us with an opportunity to heal the hurt of others. We just need to recognize the opportunity and give as much love as we can.
8. Love is contagious, so spread as much as you can.
9. During difficult times, people's true colors

will show. You will be surprised who really cares about you and who doesn't.

10. If someone hurts you, ask God to forgive them.

So, in closing, I found out how much God loves us all, and if you pray to Him, He will always help you no matter what you're going through. The same way the Lord took control of the wheel and guided me to safety, the Lord has taken control of my life and is guiding me to a cure. About miracle number three: It's been one month since my surgery. According to the doctors, my tumor should have grown two centimeters by now without treatment. I had an MRI last Wednesday, and to the surprise of my surgeon, there was no tumor growth since surgery. Once again, thank you, Lord, for stopping this tumor. Thank you all for listening, and I want to thank everyone that has prayed for me to recover. PRAYER DOES WORK.

Today I am being baptized on my twelve-year wedding anniversary. One of many blessings.

Open Letter to President Bill Clinton

Dear Mr. President,

I am, according to all the expert physicians, a terminally ill cancer patient with an "incurable" brain tumor. I was given seventeen weeks to live in November of 1995. You may be wondering how I am writing this letter from my grave. Let me explain it to you.

When all the so-called experts threw in the towel and gave me up for a goner, I prayed that God would guide me to a cure. I believe that He has. I now know that my mission in life is to prove to the world, and especially to you and Congress, that it is possible to cure deadly cancer by natural means. I'm living proof of that.

I know it doesn't go over nicely with the medical establishment, but that's their problem, not mine. I am alive for a couple of reasons: First, to bring *hope to the hopeless* cases like me that the doctors just give up on. Second, to bring change to the medical establishment and insurance companies. I know these are astronomical goals. The doctors in this country must stop feeling threatened by naturopathic doctor consultants like Dr. Dante Ruccio, who helped guide me to recovery.

I think it is time that we pass some kind of legislation that gives a person, not the doctors, the power to make one's own healthcare decisions. I have been unsuccessful to even have a radiologist document on my MRI report the fact that I have been treated with shark cartilage. They will document the fact that a person is treated with chemo or radiation, but somehow, they feel threatened and afraid of giving shark cartilage the credibility it deserves.

What are they so afraid of? Could it be that they will have to admit they've been wrong all these years? People will discover the truth that those modalities of treatment are worthless in treating brain cancer. If my suffering and experience could change one thing, I wish it would be that new laws could be passed to allow people to empower themselves. Let us choose our own treatment and have the insurance companies pay. Especially, when you have proven that it works.

Mr. President, it is a shame that a proven treatment for brain tumors such as shark cartilage, with an eighty to ninety percent success rate, is shunned by the medical establishment, while other treatments that have a zero percent cure rate are so widely accepted.

How could I change this? How could one person make a difference? Please remember, while all the experts argue about the effectiveness of shark cartilage, people are being diagnosed every day with this deadly malignant brain tumor and given a death sentence of a few months to a year with conventional treatment. People need to be informed, educated, and then allowed to make their own educated decision.

The Explanation

I was told that I belonged to a subset of patients with this glioma that could have a clinical course such as mine. I was told that I probably fit the subset of patients with primary gliomas who do very well in spite of no treatment after surgery. I was told that I fit in this category of patients who are younger than forty-five with tumors of the frontal lobe, usually male. Since I have done extensive research on my diagnosis, I knew this explanation was totally unacceptable. I began to search to find where this theory originated. I began to contact oncologists and neurosurgeons. I asked them if they were aware of such a subset of patients as explained to me. Some of the responses I received are as follows:

- "It is very unlikely that a right frontal lobe patient would be tumor free for two years after diagnosis without follow-up treatment."
- "It would be very unusual for a patient with grade IV astrocytoma or glioblastoma to be alive without signs of the tumor growing two years after surgery and no other treatment."
- "It is certainly possible, but a rare event, that a tumor of this type is completely resected and does not recur."
- "Although the prognosis for this tumor is dismal, every neurologist knows a patient who bucks the odds for unknown reasons. I know of no subset, just one lucky patient."

- "Anything is possible in medicine, but the situation you describe must be extraordinarily rare. I have seen hundreds of cases of this disease and have not seen such a case. In general, young patients with glioblastomas do better. However, in some reports of long-term survival in GM patients, the original diagnosis was found to be incorrect on later pathologic review."

My diagnosis, which I checked in three different pathology departments, all revealed a glioblastoma multiforme grade IV. I even sent my tissue sample for DNA analysis to make sure the tissue on the slide was mine and not some kind of mix-up.

Only one doctor said yes, and I could read about it in the journal Neurosurgery, volume 34, February 1994, pages 213–220. This article is entitled, "Long-Term Survival in Patients with Malignant Astrocytoma." Now that I knew where this theory came from, I went to the University of Miami Medical Library and read this article. I knew that if I read the article, it would prove that I did not belong to this subset of patients the doctor was talking about. Long-term survival was defined as a patient with a grade III or grade IV astrocytoma who lived at least thirty-six months after diagnosis.

All of these patients, not some, had been prospectively entered into a variety of nonrandomized treatment protocols, including conventional and experimental chemotherapy, interstitial radiation, interstitial hyperthermia, and a various combination of these modalities.

If you read the comments made by Kurt A. Jaeckle of Houston, Texas, it was confirmed that long-term survivors were more likely to be less than forty years old. I am forty-five years old.

They were more likely to have undergone repeated surgery. I only had one surgery.

The number of younger patients to have repeated surgery was significantly greater. This is partly why younger patients live longer.

Long-term survivors were more likely to have received adequate radiotherapy (more than 60 Gy). I never did radiotherapy.

They're more likely to have lower-grade tumors. I had a high-grade IV GBM.

And they're more likely to have received chemotherapy with nitrosourea. I never received chemotherapy of any kind.

No mention was made about the tumors being in the frontal lobe.

Long-term survival is supposedly relative to aggressive and thorough management. I did not receive any management other than the BeneFin shark cartilage.

In fact, nearly 60 percent of the patients underwent repeated surgery, and 78 percent received radiation and chemotherapy in addition to the best surgical procedure. This means that only 22 percent of the patients did not receive all three treatments. On page 214 it states the median survival time after repeated surgery was nine months. All the patients did either chemotherapy, radiation, surgery, or some type of experimental drug regimen.

From this data, the prototype of the long-term survivor with malignant astrocytoma appears to be a young patient, usually a woman, not a man as was suggested, with anaplastic astrocytoma, which is a lower grade than the glioblastoma multiforme grade IV I had. Even with this aggressive approach, on page 215, it says the median survival with grade IV is fourteen months.

Long-term survivors also had a good postoperative

Karnofsky Performance Status, the minimal residual tumor on a postoperative MRI. I had a residual moderate mass effect on postoperative MRI. They received subsequent radiotherapy (more than 60 Gy), chemotherapy with a nitrosourea, and remained in good enough condition to withstand repeat surgery at recurrence. I had no radiotherapy, no chemotherapy, and as of yet, have only had one surgery.

In the entire series of 289 patients, 58 patients lived more than thirty-six months from the time of diagnosis, a 20 percent survival rate. Of the 58 patients, a large percentage, 70.6 percent or 41 patients, underwent repeated surgery; 63.7 percent received 60 Gy radiation therapy. Almost three-fourths had been exposed to nitrosourea chemotherapy (72.4 percent).

This does not sound anything like the subset I belonged to. I did not see that I had anything in common with this group of patients. It was obvious that the doctor was reaching for straws.

The only reason I am alive is because I have been doing an all-natural treatment that is not recognized by the modern medical establishment.

The doctor did not accept the fact that the shark cartilage BeneFin product is what has been keeping me alive up until now.

Since the doctor refuses to accept the effectiveness of the shark cartilage, he wants to find some other reason other than it, to explain why I was still alive.

I was given only seventeen weeks to live back in October 1995. They were pretty sure of my outcome then, and no one ever mentioned any subset to me then.

In conclusion, what you have to ask yourself is, what is the median survival rate for a group of individuals that have no treatment at all?

I think the following data provides information on the real subgroup that I belong to.

The following information was acquired through the internet and from:

Patrick J. Kelly, MD, FACDS, Professor and Chairman Department of Neurological Surgery at New York University Medical Center

Grade IV

Grade IV astrocytoma (frequently referred to as glioblastomas or glioblastoma multiforme) is the most malignant variety of these tumors. Mitoses are frequently noted by the pathologist as the surgical specimen is examined. Mitosis is the cellular process by which cells divide, where one cell becomes two. In addition, regions of necrosis (dead tissue) are also noted where the tumor has grown so fast that parts of it have outpaced its blood supply. These tumors induce the formation of new but abnormal blood vessels, which, when identified, are also important in establishing the diagnosis.

Prognosis

The grade IV astrocytoma has the worst prognosis:

- **Seventeen weeks average (mean) survival after diagnosis without treatment.**
- Thirty weeks average survival with biopsy followed by radiation therapy.
- Thirty-seven weeks average survival following surgical removal of most of the tumor tissue component of the tumor and radiation therapy and fifty-one weeks

average survival following stereotactic volumetric resection of the tumor of the tissue component and radiation therapy.

A funny thing happened to me on my way to my fourth opinion of my pathology. I took my slide and my original report to a major university for yet another opinion. Many of my friends have asked me why I keep sending my slides to be reexamined. I tell them it is because I am my worst critic. If I am to be making any claims as to the effectiveness of shark cartilage, I have to be 150 percent convinced that my diagnosis was correct and my treatment has worked. That is the reason for my obsession with my diagnosis.

I walked into this office and asked for a second opinion. After it was examined by two pathologists, one of them being a neuropathologist, I was told that they agreed with the original report—glioblastoma multiforme grade IV. She wanted to know why I wanted a report if they agreed and I already had a report. I told her, as you know, a glioblastoma grade IV is a deadly tumor and twenty months have passed and I was still alive with no conventional treatment. She said she wanted to take another look at it. I didn't understand what the hold-up was because I was told the report was done and it just needed to be signed. She told the other pathologist that I was the patient and twenty months have elapsed since the first report and that I had not done any treatment. At that point, he decided not to sign the report that was ready for his signature. Instead, I was told that they wanted to show it to another pathologist and that I could pick it up the next day.

I immediately realized that by telling them that my outcome was favorable, their opinion had become biased. I suspected they would change their mind about the diagnosis because no one is supposed to be alive with glioblastoma grade IV twenty months later with no conventional treatment. This pathologist later spoke to me in his office and explained to me that he believed this may be a juvenile pilocytic astrocytoma. He wrote in his report that the fact that this patient has done well suggests that the tumor was more benign than it looked morphologically. He said that he had reservations about the original diagnosis, but that he did see necrosis and mitosis along with other features consistent with a glioblastoma.

He also admitted that when he was told I was doing better than expected after so long without any treatment, it raised a red flag. He was under the impression that since I did not do any conventional treatment, I didn't do any treatment at all. I told him that I have done a treatment, it just wasn't the conventional treatment of radiation and chemotherapy. I explained to him that I have been treated with the help of Dr. Ruccio, a naturopathic doctor consultant, and I went into detail about the theory behind the anti-angiogenic property of the shark cartilage. I wish I would have had a camera to capture the expression on his face. He looked at me as if I had just landed on Earth from planet Mars.

He had no idea what I was talking about and thereby totally disregarded anything I was saying as a possible explanation for my recovery. Since my treatment was foreign and unknown to him, I believe he began to look at the only possible explanation in his mind, which was a juvenile pilocytic astrocytoma, which is a relatively benign tumor that is often cured with surgery alone. Since this is the only brain tumor that can be cured with surgery alone and that was the only treatment I did, he must have concluded that this must be the only logical explanation for what I had.

I believe he began to search for anything on the slide that even resembled any characteristics of a juvenile pilocytic astrocytoma. I believe this theory was really reaching for straws. First of all, juvenile pilocytic is found primarily in children. It is a common tumor of childhood, although it rarely occurs in adults.

It most frequently occurs in the cerebellum; my tumor was in the right frontal lobe. It is surrounded by a capsule-like cyst. In my surgical report my surgeon wrote, "Although the MRI had the appearance of a cystic tumor, it was indeed solid throughout." This pathologist wrote that the tumor's appearance on the MRI was consistent with a juvenile pilocytic and not a glioblastoma multiforme.

Glioblastoma may also appear as a cyst on MRIs. Since when are diagnoses made by the appearance of the MRI, anyhow? Isn't it the job of the pathologist to examine the specimen and, according to what types of cells and features are seen under the microscope, that determines the ultimate diagnosis? In taking all of the bias and hindsight of knowing the outcome of a particular case into consideration, I believe this opinion was contaminated by the information I gave the pathologist. Therefore, I disregarded this report and continued to search for uncontaminated and unbiased reports. I have a friend who has worked many years with a pathologist, and he sent my slide to another pathologist after this episode and he said without question it was a glioblastoma grade IV. I did not get a report because it was unofficial.

In summary, to date, I have had my pathology checked five times. Four have said it was a glioblastoma multiforme grade IV, while the fifth also said it was a GBM grade IV, until he found out the fact that I have somehow overcome the diseases by unconventional means, and then he changed his mind. When one is totally convinced that what he is seeing is impossible, they will see just about anything in a slide to justify the outcome of the patient. He said he spotted Rosenthal fibers, which I believe he said are present with a juvenile pilocytic, yet no one else saw them.

Also, he mentioned piloid astrocytes (which I believe are the cells found in a pilocytic tumor) were not noted in this examination. If you don't find piloid astrocytes, doesn't that rule out juvenile pilocytic astrocytoma? He also mentioned the tumor was of low to medium cellularity, when the others said it was dense cellularity. He said many of the cells have the appearance of oligodendrocytes which the other report stated that definite areas of oligodendroglioma are not noted.

The other reports mentioned that the tumor was densely cellular, with mitotic figures, endothelial proliferation, and necrosis. All of this indicates a glioblastoma multiforme grade IV. These are features that he mentioned that he saw, but did not put it on the report. This examination, in my opinion, was very wishy-washy. "Well, it could be this, but it must be that" type of report.

When I told him that the report really didn't say anything, he chuckled. After doing some research on the internet on the appearance of a juvenile pilocytic astrocytoma on an MRI, I concluded that my MRI did not look anything like a pilocytic tumor. In a juvenile pilocytic, the classic feature is what they call the "mural nodule." The margin (lining) of the cyst does not enhance. The enhancement is limited to the "mural nodule."

I am not a radiologist, but I have eyes, and my tumor did not have a "mural nodule" and did enhance throughout the tumor. Glioblastoma multiforme is noted most frequently in the frontal lobe where mine was. It can appear as either a well-circumscribed globular mass or a more diffused mass lesion. The tumor is usually solid, although cysts may be present. My surgeon said that the tumor was indeed solid throughout.

Also, I did not experience any of the symptoms associated with juvenile pilocytic, such as headache, nausea, vomiting. I only felt fatigue and numbness in my left hand. Also, when diagnosing a juvenile pilocytic, pathologically there must be the absence of aggressive features. Meaning there must be no necrosis, no mitosis, both of which were noted in my pathology.

My question is how anyone could confuse the most malignant and fastest-growing tumor of all glioblastoma multiforme grade IV with a juvenile pilocytic astrocytoma, a childhood tumor and the least harmful of all brain tumors, which are known to be mostly benign with a good prognosis. Is it possible that because of my innocence and honesty I have played right into the medical establishment's hands? Could this be a way to explain away the effectiveness of shark cartilage? I don't know. I do know one thing: I made a mistake in mentioning that I was on this type of treatment.

Next time, I will say nothing so as not to contaminate the opinion of the pathologist. I do not think this opinion was credible, seeing how the pathologist was using hindsight and playing Monday-night quarterback. Anyone can look at a patient almost two years later and say that because he is not dead, his tumor must be more benign than it looks morphologically. What about the possibility that the shark cartilage was working? Oh no, that was not even taken into consideration. I plan to send my sample one last time to the Mayo Clinic to get an official report.

References

Cohen, M. E., and P. K. Duffner *Brain Tumors in Children*. New York: Raven Press, 1984.

Dohrmann, G. J., J. R. Farwell, and J. T. Flannery. "Glioblastoma multiforme in children." *J. Neurosurg* 44 (1976): 442–448.

Letter to the Insurance Company

If everything that has happened to me was to mean something, I felt that my experience had to bring about some positive changes. One area where I would like to see those changes was in how the insurance companies treat patients that do not believe in conventional medicine.

I felt that people who were taking charge of their own healthcare decisions were being discriminated against. I was being pressured into doing a treatment I didn't believe in simply because of financial concerns. Many cancer patients will find themselves choosing between a treatment that is covered by the insurance company and one that is not. In some cases where the conventional medical treatments show no hope of a cure, I believe the insurance companies should pay for an alternative treatment. Especially when that treatment has shown success in the past. If you are paying your premiums on time, you should not be forced to do a treatment you do not believe in. I attempted to change this practice by writing to my insurance company and placing a claim for my cancer treatment. The following is the letter I sent to my insurance carrier:

June 4, 1997

Insured: Jimmy Blanco

Dear Plan Administrator:

In October of 1995, I was diagnosed with a highly malignant brain tumor known as glioblastoma multiforme grade IV. Surgery was performed. The doctors estimated that I had seventeen weeks to live after surgery and advised me to undergo chemotherapy and radiation treatments, which, by my doctors' own admission, offered no chance of remission. I had DNA testing and pathology checked three times to make sure there were no mistakes.

Rather than accept the hopeless situation that was presented to me by the doctors, I decided to take a nutritional approach and began working with Dr. Dante Ruccio, a naturopathic doctor consultant located in Newark, New Jersey. He is a pioneer in this field and is an advocate in the use of shark cartilage to combat cancer and other diseases.

Over the past nineteen months, I have been using the shark cartilage BeneFin product. Obviously, I have by far surpassed the four months doctors gave me to live, and to the complete surprise and amazement of these doctors, the MRIs show no sign of the tumor recurring.

By choosing shark cartilage over chemotherapy and radiation treatments, your company has saved significant sums of money on doctors, hospitals, and treatments, while at the same time, my once hopeless situation is looking brighter.

You and I know that those treatments do not work in curing glioblastoma multiforme grade IV. At best it would have made me sicker and cause me many other problems that do not exist and may cause me to be hospitalized and have further surgeries.

I could cite several cases where that is exactly what occurred. They were my friends. Chemotherapy radiation and gamma knife did not work for them. One has since passed away after five surgeries, two gamma knife treatments, and radiation treatments in less than a year. Another passed away three months after diagnosis because he refused those treatments and did not attempt the shark cartilage. The other endured surgery, radiation, chemo, and the gamma knife twice. After all of that, she was sent home to die, paralyzed. After conventional medicine gave up on her, she started an alternative treatment by Dr. Recio from Spain and the BeneFin shark cartilage with Dr. Ruccio. This was almost two years ago and she was alive and walking.

Another option for me might have been the gamma knife, which is not a cure but another worthless option that can easily cost one hundred thousand dollars. Now that you know I am a survivor nineteen months after a decree of only seventeen weeks to live, you will be able to implement cost-cutting, ground-breaking options for your customers.

I know you would not want me to be obligated to do a treatment that does not give me any hope of survival. You would choose the treatment that when studied, reviewed, and prayed about for yourself, reflected the hope of living.

The total expense which improves your bottom line is only $12,769.31 over the past nineteen months for this product's usage.

Without continued use of the shark cartilage, there is a likelihood, according to Dr. Ruccio, that the tumor will reappear. If that occurs, the expense of hospitalization, additional surgeries, and treatment will be astronomical.

Although the cost of the shark cartilage is relatively low when compared to conventional treatment, it is an expense which I will not be able to sustain for an extended period of time; furthermore, it is an expense that I believe should be covered under my plan.

Shark cartilage has an eighty to ninety percent success rate with brain tumors, compared with a zero percent cure rate from chemotherapy, gamma knife, and radiation.

Currently, nineteen months after surgery, I am still alive. Talk to any oncologist—he will tell you it is extraordinarily rare to live nineteen months with a glioblastoma multiforme grade IV, with or without chemotherapy and radiation treatment.

This is terrific! Shark cartilage is working and keeping my tumor in check. I have a friend who has thirty years in the insurance business and he explained loss ratios to me for insurance providers. One of your agents mentioned that, actually, the company knows how much they will spend and how many of the same kind of people with my type of tumor will impact their profits. He also said that providers like to pay claims when it will be in their best interest, help the patient, and sincerely help their bottom line. He said a provider paying for a major illness not much more than the annual premiums is rare.

As you may be aware, one of your major competitors announced in 1993 it would reimburse patients for an alternative program shown to reverse heart disease without drugs or surgery. From a business perspective, their decision very likely saved the company money over the long term.

Advancements are being made in the naturopathic approach that in my case, and in others like it, could save your company money as well.

While writing my book, which is now completed and soon to be with the publisher, I have dug far under the surface of conventional medicine. My book, *Hope for the*

Hopeless, will touch and change for the better many people's lives.

The challenge for healthcare policymakers and federal regulators is to ensure the public's access to the most effective treatments available.

Now and in the future, patients will have recourse when it can be shown that their practitioners, and/or providers', paid treatment offers no clinical or psychological benefit. By the same token, patients with debilitating, severe, or chronic illnesses should be guaranteed a right to insurance-covered alternative therapy they believe offers them relief or a cure that is reasonable and soon to be customary.

As you know, many physicians are neither trained in nor possess a degree in alternative healing. Times are changing, and patients will have the right to see knowledgeable healthcare professionals that will be vital to his or her care.

The shark cartilage is vital to my future health, and I trust that you will seriously consider my claim. Enclosed is your claim form and copies of receipts for BeneFin shark cartilage product used to date.

I want to thank you in advance for the assistance and payment of my claim. Thank you for being here for me and helping me stay away from the knife and antiquated treatment. I look forward to your response.

Sincerely,
Jimmy Blanco[8]

---

[8] Jimmy never heard back from the White House, and his requested claim to cover the cost of shark cartilage was denied by his health insurance company.

List of Helpful Organizations and Websites

American Cancer Society, www.cancer.org

American clinical trials, www.clinicaltrials.gov

Private clinical trials, www.centerwatch.com

European clinical trials, www.clinicaltrialsregister.eu

National Center for Biotechnology Information of the NIH, www.ncbi.nlm.nih.gov

NIH National Cancer Institute, www.cancer.gov

American Association of Neurological Surgeons, www.aans.org
Patients can find a board-certified neurosurgeon, watch educational videos.

Preston Robert Tisch Brain Tumor Center at Duke University, https://tischbraintumorcenter.duke.edu/

Cousins Center for Psychoneuroimmunology at the Semel Institute for Neuroscience and Human Behavior at UCLA, www.semel.ucla.edu/cousins

UCLA Mindful Awareness Research Center, www.uclahealth.org/marc/

American Board of Naturopathic Oncology, www.fabno.org

Oncology Association of Naturopathic Physicians, www.oncanp.org
Patients can find an NP.

Human Nature Natural Health, Ian D. Bier, N.D., Ph.D., L.Ac., FABNO, https://www.humannaturenaturalhealth.com/dr-bier

EuroMed Foundation, www.euromedfoundation.com

Dedicated to an integrative cancer treatment philosophy with an emphasis on strengthening the immune system.

Glioblastoma Research Organization, www.gbmresearch.org

Glioblastoma Foundation, www.glioblastomafoundation.org
They help to match patients to clinical trials.

National Brain Tumor Society, www.braintumor.org

Brain Tumour Foundation of Canada, www.braintumour.ca

National Coalition for Cancer Survivorship, www.canceradvocacy.org

Mayo Clinic, www.mayoclinic.org

Imerman Angels, www.imermanangels.org
A free one-on-one cancer support program.

Coping with Cancer **Magazine**, www.copingmag.com

Radical Remission Project, www.radicalremission.com
A place to share and read stories of extraordinary remission from terminal diseases.

Chris Beat Cancer, www.chrisbeatcancer.com
Find nutritional cancer coaching and great information from super cancer–survivor Chris Wark.

Physicians Committee for Responsible Medicine, www.pcrm.org

The Exam Room **Podcast**
Subscribe on GooglePlay, Apple Podcasts, Stitcher, or Spotify.

World Health Organization, www.who.int/health-topics/cancer

The Truth about Cancer: A Global Quest,
go.thetruthaboutcancer.com
A nine-part docu-series on cancer.

**Find updated resources, book recommendations, and more online at www.hopeforthehopelessbook.com.
You can also find the book on social media by searching @hopeforthehopelessbook.**

Recommended Reading

The Biology of Belief by Dr. Bruce Lipton

Chris Beat Cancer: A Comprehensive Plan for Healing Naturally by Chris Wark

Embrace, Release, Heal: An Empowering Guide to Talking About, Thinking About and Treating Cancer by Leigh Fortson

Radical Remission: Surviving Cancer Against All Odds by Dr. Kelly Turner

Radical Hope: 10 Key Healing Factors from Exceptional Survivors of Cancer & Other Diseases by Dr. Kelly Turner

How Not to Die: Discover the Foods Scientifically Proven to Prevent and Reverse Disease by Dr. Michael Greger

Beating Cancer with Nutrition by Dr. Patrick Quillin

A Holistic Protocol for the Immune System by Scott J. Gregory

Heinerman's Encyclopedia of Healing Herbs & Spices by John Heinerman

Stop Feeding Your Cancer by Dr. John Kelly

What to Eat During Cancer Treatment by Barbara L. Grant and Jeanne Besser

Raw Vegetable Juices by N. W. Walker, DSc

There Is a River: The Story of Edgar Cayce by Thomas Sugrue

St. Francis of Assisi: A Biography by Omer Englebert

Angels in My Hair by Lorna Byrne

The Mushin Way to Peak Performance: The Path to Productivity, Balance, and Success by Michael Veltri

Healthy at Last: A Plant-Based Approach to Preventing and Reversing Diabetes and Other Chronic Illnesses by Eric Adams

Acknowledgments

To my mother, Elizabeth. You are the strongest, most coura-geous, resilient, and unrelentingly optimistic and bubbly person I've ever met. You've done everything for us. There's no way to repay you, except to send you on an all-expenses-paid vacation to Spain one day. I'll work on that. Love you!

To my soul mate, best friend, and incredible husband, Ron. Thank you for being my anchor in the storm. You've helped make my dreams come true in every way possible. I'll get you a lobster dinner after this.

To my crazy bears, Nicholas and Desiree. Thank you for choos-ing me to be your mom. I love you to infinity and beyond! You can accomplish anything you set your hearts to in this life, but I hope you set your hearts to being happy and kind and silly and weird. Let's have a dance party!

Thanks to Ronald and Valerie for being my second parents and being among the most supportive and loving people I know.

To Lorna and Pearl Byrne for their kindness and grace in grant-ing this very special interview.

To my forever Sensei, Michael Veltri, for his unstoppable spirit, relentless positivity, integrity, and courage. It's an honor to mark you among my friends.

To the amazing Chuck Carroll, thank you for being my cheer-leader, and I'm so excited to see you changing the world for the better.

To Dr. Ian Bier, Dr. Eduardo Recio Roura, and Dr. Puneet Chandak for lending your expertise to help the readers of this book.

To Sandra Hillburn, wishing you many more years with your grandkids and those delicious mini ice cream cones.

And to my WNEW family for encouraging and supporting me. I love you guys!

And infinite thanks to every single person who chipped in and helped me make this book possible, including May Day Blanco, Daniel and Tina Gallant, Tony and Ivon Blanco, Charlie Bergeron, Dwight Henriquez and Alyssa Zamora, Jonathan DelValle, Stephanie Palacino, Dave Carty (the hardest-working guy in the biz), James Rojas, Yaima Suarez, *y todos los muchisimos!*

Gracias a mi quieridas abuelas Trinidad y Eva. Gracias a mis abuelos en el cielo, Antonio y Jorge. Thank for being one of my best friends, Pisi! (Reylo forever!) And thanks to Joanna Schaffhausen, and Deanna and Lazaro Blanco for helping me proofread parts of this book.

And of course, a very special thanks to my friend Juri Love, who God put in my path to help me get this book across the finish line. I wouldn't be here if it wasn't for you. Finally, thank you for reading this book and doing your best. I love you.

—Jamie Blanco

About the Author

A son of hard-working Cuban immigrants, Jimmy Blanco grew up on the mean streets of Newark, New Jersey, in the 1960s and '70s. He served in the army and navy before moving to Miami where he met his beautiful wife, Elizabeth. Jimmy became a respiratory therapist and was well-known and respected in South Florida medical circles.

When he got his terminal diagnosis, he felt his purpose in life had been revealed to him. He dedicated the rest of his life to proving his doctors wrong and to bringing hope to hopeless causes like himself.

Jimmy's daughter, Jamie, is an award-winning radio news producer residing in the Boston area. Jamie spent several years working to realize her father's dream of publishing his book of hope for cancer patients. Jamie enjoys nerd culture, hosts an iHeartRadio podcast called *The Hub on Hollywood*, and is now a frequent background actor in film and television.

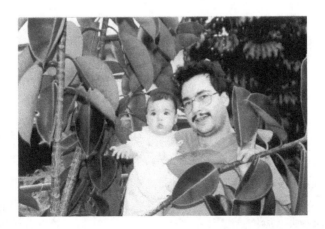

CPSIA information can be obtained
at www.ICGtesting.com
Printed in the USA
BVHW091038140622
639733BV00016B/988